T'ai Chi

for Seniors

How to Gain Flexibility, Strength, and Inner Peace

By

Sifu Philip Bonifonte

/2/

T'ai Chi
for Seniors

HOW
TO GAIN
FLEXIBILITY,
STRENGTH,
AND INNER
PEACE

By

Sifu Philip Bonifonte

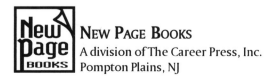

NEW PAGE BOOKS
A division of The Career Press, Inc.
Pompton Plains, NJ

T'AI CHI FOR SENIORS
EDITED AND TYPESET BY STACEY A. FARKAS
Cover design by Lu Rossman/Digi Dog Design
Printed in the U.S.A.

To order this title, please call toll-free 1-800-CAREER-1 (NJ and Canada: 201-848-0310) to order using VISA or MasterCard, or for further information on books from Career Press.

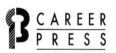

The Career Press, Inc., 220 West Parkway, Unit 12
Pompton Plains, NJ 07444
www.careerpress.com
www.newpagebooks.com

Library of Congress Cataloging-in-Publication Data

Bonifonte, Philip, 1958-
    T'ai chi for seniors : how to gain flexibility, strength, and inner peace / by
Philip Bonifonte.
        p. cm.
    Includes index.
    ISBN 1-56414-697-9 (pbk.)
        1. Tai chi for the aged. I. Title.

GV504.6.A35B66 2004
613.7'148--dc22   2003060207

Dedication

To Anthony and Michael, who have taught me to laugh at life.

To Doreen and AJ, without whose help, support, and love this book would have been impossible to write.

To my teachers over the years, both in the martial arts world and the "other" one.

To my students, wherever they are on the Path. Thank you for being both students and teachers.

To Linda Paul, for her photography.

Contents

Part I: Living in the Past
9

Part II: Living in the Present
57

Part III: Living in the Future
133

Part I

Living in
the Past

Chapter 1

What Is T'ai Chi, and Why Should I Care?

The Basics

What Is T'ai Chi?

A solitary figure moves slowly and gracefully in the early morning mist settling over the park. Her movements are relaxed, yet contain a hint of controlled power. Her posture is remarkable, appearing upright yet not stiff; she glides over the dew-covered grass in what can only be described as a gentle dance.

As you draw closer, you see her momentarily change the tempo of the dance, performing a blindingly fast kick with her right leg, then resuming her stately ballet. She ends the movements with a momentary stillness, a calm that you can almost feel. Thinking that this is one of the local college girls practicing for her dance class, you decide to approach her and ask what school she attends. Maybe the school offers ballroom lessons....

Twenty feet away, you are shocked to see that her hair has some gray in it. She turns in your direction and smiles at you...she must be at least 50. Closer still, you spy the wrinkles and laugh lines. Sixty? Her voice contains a tinkling laugh as she greets you, and you cannot help but notice that there is something about her, some type of happiness or joy; you see it in her face and the way she holds herself.

After a spirited 20-minute conversation, you are in awe. She is 72 years old! She's got a good 12 years on you, and you could not imagine being that graceful. She must have good genes. Too bad she's just visiting here. If that's what that "Tie Chee" stuff does for you, maybe you should look into it.

Welcome to the world of T'ai Chi. This little story illustrates a few important points about what T'ai Chi really is. Of course, as they say in the commercials, your mileage may vary, but one thing is certain: Practicing T'ai Chi, even at its most basic level, will bestow a more relaxed mind, calmer spirit, and flexible body, along with the improvements of how *you* feel about *yourself*. Strong and sexy? You bet.

T'ai Chi (*tie chee*), also occasionally spelled Taiji, is a system of exercises developed over a span of hundreds of years in China. Originally designed as a fighting method similar to Kung Fu, T'ai Chi has so much more to offer for today's mature adult. Starting to feel some pain in the left wrist? T'ai Chi can help. Recovering from a stroke? Yep, it can help that, too. It's great for balance problems. Too much stress in your life? That's a T'ai Chi specialty.

The exercises and movements of T'ai Chi are performed in a slow and relaxed fashion, as opposed to most Western styles of exercise. T'ai Chi is:

- Noncompetitive.
- Nonimpact.
- Highly aerobic (in the sense that you are breathing deeply).
- Wonderful for joint health.
- Useful for increasing blood oxygen levels and flow.
- Useful for decreasing high blood pressure.
- Great for increasing range of motion.
- Commonly used to reduce the effects of stress.
- A way to increase your balance and gracefulness.
- A way to meet and socialize with like-minded people your age.

T'ai Chi is perhaps the ultimate exercise for mature adults given its remarkable benefits and nonimpact, slow-speed performance.

Speaking of slow speed, I once had a student, a young lady of some athletic ability, who was cursed with the modern-day affliction of stress. She felt she had to cram as much activity as possible into her already impossible schedule. Constantly running from one appointment to the next, she actually found time to fit her introductory T'ai Chi class into her calendar. Showing up 10 minutes late with a harried expression on her face, she listened to my welcoming speech, all the while tapping her toes, and nervously watched me perform some Qigong movements (more about Qigong in coming chapters). Finally she blurted, "I have two weeks scheduled for these classes—is it going to take any longer than that?" After informing her that T'ai Chi often becomes the study of a lifetime, but that the benefits would start to appear in days or weeks, she simply shook her head and left. So much for an easy cure!

You can perform T'ai Chi just about anywhere. It's been performed on cruise ships, at picnics, in the park; it can even be done in your living room. You don't need a ton of expensive sports gear or fancy machinery. Just yourself, and a little bit of time.

In the touching movie *Pushing Hands,* an elderly T'ai Chi master, mourning the loss of his wife, feeling abandoned by his children, and out of step with modern times, begins to fall into depression. He runs away from his son's home where he's living, gets a job washing dishes in a restaurant, promptly loses the job, and ends up in jail on a civil disturbance charge. What do you think saves him? That's right— T'ai Chi. He rediscovers his strength, his appeal to the opposite sex, and his reason for living. In the end, he is happily teaching T'ai Chi at a community center, living in his own apartment, and beginning a beautiful relationship with his lady friend.

I have experienced many of these same benefits throughout my 32 years of practicing T'ai Chi, and I firmly believe that you will, too. All it takes is a little practice, a little faith, and an indomitable spirit. The fact that you've gotten to this point in life proves that you have the spirit.Congratulations! What you need now is the faith, the open mind that approaches the T'ai Chi exercises as a new challenge. Don't worry about the "practice" part—I guarantee that you'll love T'ai Chi so much, you'll want to practice all day long, maybe even for weeks!

What T'ai Chi Is Not

T'ai Chi and Yoga

Yoga, as a system of exercise for both the body and the spirit, has been popular in the West for many more years than T'ai Chi. There are truckloads of books and videotapes devoted to its many variations, and you can usually find a yoga class very easily. It is a wonderful system of stretches and breathing exercises suitable for many people.

So why don't more mature adults practice yoga? I always ask my new students if they've ever taken yoga classes before. Usually they'll answer yes, but that they couldn't twist themselves into pretzels as the instructor did, so they quit. But is that the only reason?

Sometimes it's because of the teaching style of the instructor. Some teachers are just too advanced for their beginning students, expecting them to touch the floor with their fingers while their knees are locked, or perform headstands. This is too much for most of the beginning students, who proceed to the door with as much haste as they can muster.

Sometimes it's because of false expectations on the part of the student. You heard from your friend that the new yoga instructor at the YMCA is great, that she hasn't felt this good in years, it's easy. Why not come on down and try it? You go to the class and, true to her word, your friend is bending herself into a pretzel shape, all the while chanting strange words. *This looks too hard*, you think. *Better just slip out to the aqua-aerobics class and call it a day.*

T'ai Chi is not yoga. No bending into weird, contorted shapes; no chanting. The biggest difference between the two modalities is that yoga advocates stillness while T'ai Chi seeks movement. You are constantly in motion when you perform your T'ai Chi exercises. The Taoist philosophy behind T'ai Chi (which we'll examine in detail in Chapter 11) states that movement is life and stillness is death. With yoga, at least with the popular styles such as Hatha Yoga, you strike a pose and hold it while you breathe. Sometimes the instructor even asks you to hold your breath. Do you imagine yourself turning blue? With T'ai Chi there's no holding your breath; just slow, relaxed inhales and exhales. Natural breathing. If you're not comfortable with one of the T'ai Chi positions, don't worry. You'll be moving out of it before you experience any pain.

T'ai Chi and Aerobics

Have you ever gone to the local gym or workout center and watched with growing apprehension the stick-thin girls bouncing up and down on those colorful plastic steps? The teacher has that tiny microphone in front of her mouth and is screaming out, "One, Two, three, four, and switch, two, three, four," and the other stick-girls are gleefully stepping in perfect cadence to the booming beat.

Depressing, huh?

That's aerobics. Whether you're on a treadmill, a stationary bicycle, attending a power aerobics class, or jogging on the street, you're doing aerobics. You're trying to maintain that target heart rate for the optimal length of time so your lungs get filled with oxygen. At least, that's the conventional wisdom. When I look at these folks, all I see is the pain on their faces. No Pain, No Gain. Sure.

We have a saying at my T'ai Chi school: "If there's pain, you're not using your brain."

Now, I'm a big guy. I'm 6 feet tall, and run about 220 pounds. I've been doing martial arts for more than 32 years, and I'm in excellent shape. Yet I cannot see myself doing those exercises. There's just something about looking so sweaty and pained that you're going to drop that goes against my better instincts. Yes, you get a thorough workout. Yes, you're pumping that oxygen into the blood. But that face!

You can accomplish the same thorough workout and oxygen-pumping with T'ai Chi, without any of the painful faces. Our diaphragmatic breathing techniques ensure a full, oxygen-rich cardiovascular system, without all the bouncing and sweating, not to mention the chance of getting sideswiped by a car while you're jogging, or slipping off those little colorful steps while you enviously watch the lithe instructor. To me, the choice is clear.

T'ai Chi and the New Age

This section may be difficult for some of you to take. I have nothing against anyone trying to achieve enlightenment, seeking answers to cosmic questions, or attempting to feel the vibrations from a collection of crystals. Some of what we practice in T'ai Chi, especially at the more advanced levels, seems like magic to many folks.

But T'ai Chi does not belong in this category. If anything, it should go into the history section, because the practice of these exercises goes back hundreds or, if you count Qigong exercises, thousands of years. Better yet, let's put it in the Alternative Medicine category. In Chapter 2, we'll be looking at the general health benefits that T'ai Chi offers us, and we'll go into more detail on the rehabilitative uses of T'ai Chi in Chapter 10. For now, let's just say that T'ai Chi produces some of its wonderful effects in my students after the first class.

But New Age? No, sorry. It's not in the cards.

A Short History of T'ai Chi

Unless you practice genealogy as a hobby, or become so intensely involved in T'ai Chi that it takes over your life (not that there's anything wrong with that!), a long retelling of the history of T'ai Chi would probably just serve to make you curl up in your recliner and take a nap. I'll promise to keep this brief if you promise to read it and try to understand why T'ai Chi is such a special endeavor.

Chinese history is chock-full of colorful legends, snarling dragons, and heroic figures both male and female. So it stands to reason that T'ai Chi would not be without its share. We'll start with the commonly told legend of how T'ai Chi was created.

Chang San-Feng, a Taoist priest, was practicing his martial arts movements back in 14th-century China. Finishing up, he lay down under a tree to catch a few winks. Suddenly, he was jolted awake by loud, screeching noises. Glancing around, he spotted a snake and a crane engaged in a deadly duel. The snake, coiling and uncoiling smoothly, would strike out with blinding speed at the crane, which would push this attack aside with a brush of his wing. Then the crane would strike with his beak, but the snake would just as nimbly move out of range. After the fight wore on for hours, the snake and crane finally parted, neither one victorious.

Chang had an idea, one that formed as he watched the two animals fighting. Why couldn't a human fight like that? The soft, supple movements of the snake's body and the crane's wing could be imitated, along with the fast, explosive strikes. The yin and the yang.

Happy birthday, T'ai Chi.

Of course, prior to observing this historic battle, Chang had been practicing movements that were brought to China thousands of years earlier by a gentleman named Bodhidharma ("Da Mo" in Chinese), a Buddhist monk from India. He created a series of exercises for the monks of the Shaolin Temple when he saw their wretched physical and spiritual condition. The basic principles and techniques of movement later coalesced into what would become Qigong.

So, to truly understand T'ai Chi, we need to learn a bit about Qigong. We'll take care of that in Chapter 3. For now, just know that Qigong and T'ai Chi are twins, that one cannot truly be said to thrive without acknowledging the other.

The Five Main Styles of T'ai Chi

Just as there are many styles of dancing, there are several styles, or schools, of T'ai Chi. Although a complete understanding of the history and evolution of T'ai Chi can be an absorbing pursuit, most of the details are of interest only to T'ai Chi scholars, so we'll touch only briefly on the subject. Just a note here: Many of T'ai Chi's origin stories can stretch the limits of believability. Realize that in 13th-century China, not everyone was well versed in the realities of life. People often would ascribe great feats to the T'ai Chi masters, feats that to our Western minds are quite impossible. But the Chinese have always had a penchant for creating legends out of mortal acts, so read what you will into the more colorful legends.

Chen Style

Chen Style is often said to be the original T'ai Chi, named after General Chen Wangting of Chen Village in China. General Chen lived in the 17th century and developed this style when he needed a combination of soft and hard movements for his troops to employ in battle. It is said that he heard of the infamous snake and crane battle that started the whole T'ai Chi ball rolling and built upon that foundation. General Chen kept the secrets of Chen Style within his family for many years, until the appearance of Yang Luchan (the section "Yang Style" that follows will examine what happened then).

Chen Style tends to be more martial in its approach to the exercises, with lower stances, some fast movements interspersed throughout the forms, and stomping of the feet. Although it is usually conceded to be the original style of T'ai Chi, it is harder to find Chen practitioners in the West, and as a result, it is only second or third in popularity. This is not the best style to attempt if you are at all unsure of your physical abilities.

Yang Style

Yang Style is perhaps the most common form, or style, of T'ai Chi in the West. Nine times out of 10, if you take a T'ai Chi class at the recreation center or YMCA, you'll be learning Yang Style. Yang Style is said to be the invention of Yang Luchan from the Henan Village in the 1800s, who, as a boy, covertly watched the Chen family practice their T'ai Chi at night. He would then practice on his own, adding and modifying movements as he saw fit. Caught one day and ordered to spar with the Chen students, he soundly beat them all. Thus began the teaching of Yang Style T'ai Chi, which was subsequently passed down to Yang Luchan's son and grandson, who further developed the style.

The characteristics of Yang Style are slow, large, graceful movements that flow from one pose to the next, an upright posture, and a slight bend to the legs. Properly taught, this is the easiest style for the mature student to learn. The basic T'ai Chi exercises that you will be learning in Chapter 7 are based mainly on Yang Style movements.

Wu/Hao Style

The third oldest style, Wu/Hao is seen as having the smallest, most refined movements of the five styles. Created by Wu Yuxiang, a student of Yang T'ai Chi (who also became a student of Chen Style), Wu/Hao Style is perhaps the most meditative of all T'ai Chi styles. (The two names for this style come from the fact that Hao Weizhen is the man actually credited with developing this style. Additionally, there is another style named Wu Style, so these two names serve to differentiate the styles.) Wu/Hao is the fourth most popular style in the West.

Wu Style

This style is marked by a slight lean forward, higher stances, and rapid execution of small movements. Often believed to be a variation of Yang Style, Wu is the third most practiced style today.

Sun Style

Sun Style is a fairly recent addition to the T'ai Chi world. It is a blending of several styles, characterized by fast hand and slow leg movements, and is probably the least known and practiced style in the West.

So, Which Style Should I Do?

Chances are, you won't have much of a choice. T'ai Chi, while becoming more popular every day, is not yet as ubiquitous as McDonalds. You may just have to settle for whatever the local school teaches.

Don't despair. Remember, Yang Style is the most prevalent style in the United States, so you'll more than likely be studying that. It actually works to your advantage, because Yang is the easiest and least martial-like of all the styles. But don't be turned off by the other styles. All T'ai Chi movements share certain basic principles that can greatly benefit seniors, as long as they are properly taught and adapted.

Chapter 2

Hey, That Feels Good!

The Benefits of Practicing T'ai Chi

Much like any other mode of exercise or mental stimulation, T'ai Chi gives to the practitioner only what the practitioner gives to it. The historical benefits sought from T'ai Chi in ancient China were perhaps different from what we in the West are seeking today, but this fact makes it no less important to study and practice diligently.

The benefits of T'ai Chi can be broken down into three main areas:

1. Physical.

2. Mental.

3. Spiritual.

We will begin this chapter with what is perhaps the most impressive and commonly seen benefit: the physical improvement in health.

Physical Benefits of T'ai Chi Practice

T'ai Chi cultivates health benefits beyond those studied by Western medicine. T'ai Chi conditions the sleeves between muscles and nerves (the films that separate and support the organs) known as the fascia. The acupuncture meridians (energy pathways) of Chinese medicine run through the fascia. By conditioning these boundary layers between tissues, T'ai Chi reduces chemical cross-linking, or cellular rust. Move it or lose it, the Taoists say. The turning of the trunk flexes the spine, producing some of the same benefits as twists in yoga (improved spinal flexibility, release of tension on the perispinal muscles, alleviating imbalances that can lead to back pain while improving blood flow to the discs). And similar to yoga, T'ai Chi conditions the psoas, that deep muscle of balance that underlies the lower abdominal organs and mediates the relationship of the spine to the pelvis and legs. Proper T'ai Chi practice places certain demands on the body: The sinking of the weight, over time, tells the legs to add muscle and bone mass, while the turning of the body, in conjunction with deep abdominal breathing, "wrings out" the organs, flushing blood out as they're compressed and allowing it to flow back in when the movement compresses another part of the torso. This flexing and unflexing reduces pockets of stagnation in the various organ systems.

Physical Strength

Physical strength peaks in the mid-20s, declines modestly to age 50, and steeply thereafter. Studies show a loss of one-third of lower extremity strength by age 70. In advanced age, few people are able to stand on one leg for more than a few seconds. Premature decline need not be the case. T'ai Chi exercises all the joints and major muscle groups in a slow, rhythmic, mindful way, priming the body for whatever demands the day may make. Leg strength increases with practice, which pays off with every step you take, every time you stand in line, every time you climb a flight of stairs. Your joints stay loose and flexible, so everyday chores around the house and garden don't take as much out of you. When you practice T'ai Chi in the morning, it's easier to move for the rest of the day and concentrate on what you have to do. You waste less energy and attention on body static, so you have the stamina to ride out crazy days and long hours at work and still have something left for your family, your mate, your art. T'ai Chi is for anyone who wants to move with greater strength, grace, and ease as they get older.

In the United States, studies have shown that even people in their 70s and 80s can learn a simplified series of T'ai Chi forms, and benefit tremendously. Study subjects show a marked decrease in injurious falls, reduction in blood pressure, and improved measures of balance and confidence.

Stress Reduction

Stress is competing demands, overabundant choices, too much to do in too little time. Stress is modern living, the American way. Chronic stress is bad because it makes the body focus on short-term emergencies, at the expense of long-term regeneration. Chronic stress undermines the body's ability to fix itself.

The stress response is designed to get you out of immediate danger: Your body mobilizes energy and delivers it where it's needed most. Glucose and amino acids are released from storage in your fat cells, your liver, and your muscles. Heart rate, blood pressure, and breathing rate all go up. Blood supply is shunted from the organs (except for the heart and lungs) to the skeletal muscles. Pain is suppressed, and the mind achieves a peculiar clarity. Digestion shuts down, regenerative processes are put on hold, reproductive urges and capabilities dwindle, and, for some as yet unexplained reason, the body starts actively dismantling the immune system.

That the stress response itself can become harmful makes a certain amount of sense when you examine the things that occur in reaction to stress. They are the sorts of costly things your body has to do to respond effectively in an emergency. If you experience every day as an emergency, you will pay the price.

If you constantly mobilize energy at the cost of energy storage, you will never store any surplus energy. You will fatigue more rapidly, and your risk of developing a form of diabetes will increase. The consequences of chronically overactivating your cardiovascular system are similarly damaging: If your blood pressure rises to 180/140 when you are sprinting away from a lion, you are being adaptive, but if it is 180/140 every time you see the mess in your teenager's bedroom, you could be heading for cardiovascular disease.

This is the bodily cost of chronic stress; life as we know it. We make it hard for our bodies to fix themselves. Anything we can do to dissipate stress is time and energy well spent. T'ai Chi is a great way to reduce stress. The mental focus of the mind leading the movement; thinking only of the movement; the slow, flowing shifts of balance; the regular, deep breathing; the harmonious turning of the limbs; and the circular openings and closings of the T'ai Chi form make it one of the best stress reducers available.

Unlike so many other physical exercises practiced today, T'ai Chi does not harm the body. Its slow, gentle movements are designed to soothe rather than stress, and place no undue strain upon the muscles, joints, or connective tissues. Even walking can be a higher impact exercise than T'ai Chi. This isn't to say that the other forms of exercise are wrong—they just may be wrong for *you*.

In the many forms of T'ai Chi practice are found some that can equal the toughest aerobic workouts in terms of perspiration and muscle stretching. More commonly found in the West are the softer forms, performed slowly and with upright posture. In between, you can probably find a style of T'ai Chi that is perfect for you and your needs.

Increased Energy

My students often remark how energized they feel after a class, and in one way this is due to the simple fact that they are moving. So much of our society today is devoted to the sofa and easy chair—computers and television are probably the two biggest culprits here. So, T'ai Chi offers a safe way to get moving again, and to regain that mobility and healthy glow.

Coordination and Circulation

The effects of T'ai Chi upon the body's coordination are well known, and will benefit both the seasoned athlete and the "armchair warrior." Whether you are golfing in Florida or lugging the groceries in from the car in Pennsylvania, T'ai Chi will help energize you and allow you to move in the most efficient, safest, and ergonomically correct fashion.

Another physical benefit of T'ai Chi is that of massaging the feet. Ever had a foot massage? Felt good, right? T'ai Chi massages the bottom of the feet, stimulating the acupuncture points grouped there, and leading to general circulatory and balance improvement. According the Traditional Chinese Medicine theory, the bottom of the feet contain energy pathways, or meridians, that lead to all of the body's internal organs. So, in a sense, you are massaging your organs by gently moving back and forth on your feet.

Listening to Your Body

The theory of Chinese medicine will be examined in more detail in Chapter 12. Another physical benefit accrued from T'ai Chi practice is that of learning to "listen" to the body. By this, I don't mean listening for the various bodily sounds, those snaps, crackles, and pops that we all have, but to learn how to feel and interpret the various sensations produced from T'ai Chi movements and equate them with your overall level of health. Here's an example from one of my students. Jane (all names have been changed), 57, came to my class one rainy day in May and told me that she was a mess. "I can't get through my day at work because of the pain I have. I've heard T'ai Chi can help. Can it?"

Upon further questioning, I discovered that Jane had been living with her pain for more than 12 years. The most upsetting thing to her was the sudden onset of the pain, with no warning. She felt she could deal with it, if she had time to prepare herself mentally. The cause of her pain, arthritis and fibromyalgia, was not important at this point—her mechanism for recognizing and dealing with is was.

In the course of T'ai Chi instruction over the next three months, Jane learned many techniques for recognizing the onset of the pains, often many hours in advance of the actual event. Her T'ai Chi practice taught her to tune in to her body, to gain a new self-diagnostic tool to use in her fight against these crippling diseases. She was able to adjust her posture and her breathing, make use of meditation exercises, and set herself both physically and mentally for the coming battle. As a result, Jane was able to more easily get through her day.

Personal Acceptance

When you reach a certain age, the idea of going down to the gym for a few hours begins to pale somewhat. The young crowd and the loud music contribute to a sense of unease and of not belonging. One of the most glaringly obvious problems with our Western exercise system is that health is equated with a "perfect" body. Ladies, how many times have you looked at the cover of *Cosmo* or *Vogue* and sighed with envy? Did you, at that time and place in your life, really want to look like that? Did you think that was the perfect body? Guys, same thing for us, but of course, different role models—Rambo, Arnold, and the like.

Like Popeye said, "I am what I am." Our society's obsession with thin and beautiful is a disease more insidious than arthritis. What constitutes beautiful? How thin is thin enough? The problem here is the overemphasis on the external, or yang, aspect of you. Physical beauty fades in time; the skin wrinkles; hair turns gray or falls out. So what? You're still you. T'ai Chi places great importance on the concept of balance, of finding peace in both the body and mind. How can the mind ever be happy if it is not happy with the body? T'ai Chi teaches us to accept what, and who, we are.

Losing Weight With T'ai Chi

We all want to lose weight, for whatever reason. Keeping the ideas of the previous paragraph in mind, make sure you want to lose the weight for the right reasons. Lose it for you, not for someone else. Lose it because you feel better at your target weight. Lose it because you'll be healthier. Lose it because you love yourself. But don't lose it because of what others think or say or do.

T'ai Chi helps you to lose weight in an efficient, healthy manner. It works from the inside out, bringing your peace of mind and positive self-image to bear on the weight issue. Again, this is the flaw in so many of the fad diets—they address the calories, but not the whole person. The positive attitude gained from T'ai Chi practice enables you to intelligently choose a weight-loss program and stick with it for *your* reasons. The more T'ai Chi you do, the more positive your self-image becomes, the more you want to lose the weight and look and feel better. Another aspect of T'ai Chi practice comes into play at this point. The calming effect of the movements leads to an overall calmer attitude toward life. This will serve to eliminate the nervous snacking and habitual binging that plague so many people in our society. When you are healthy and happy, you don't feel the need to overeat, or on the other hand, to deny yourself any type of food. You'll rely upon your new body/mind connection instead of food.

Posture

Your posture is perhaps one of the most important considerations in your overall health, yet it is rarely mentioned or prescribed by your doctor. Correct posture not only leads to a healthier outward appearance, but to more efficient use of oxygen by the lungs and greater blood circulation. The bones and muscles in the body will work in tandem rather than opposition, and the joints and connective tissues will be lubricated and stretched comfortably.

T'ai Chi can address postural problems stemming from stroke, arthritis, fibromyalgia, and many other afflictions.

Mental Benefits of T'ai Chi Practice

There are so many mental benefits of practicing T'ai Chi that it would take an entire book to examine them in detail, but for us, right here and right now (another Taoist concept that we'll examine later), here are a few of the most important ones.

Stress Reduction

We've already examined the effects of stress in our lives in the first part of this chapter, but just to recap, stress is a disease, beginning in the mind and transferring its effects to the body. If you can control the mind, the body will be safe.

Focus and Concentration

Ever get one of those "senior moments"? We all do. T'ai Chi can help lessen their occurrence through promoting focus in the movements of the form, and later, with sufficient practice, into our everyday lives.

Mental Stimulation

Studies have proven that the more you use your brain, the sharper it remains, much like a door hinge: If the door is in constant use, the hinges remain functional. If the door is never used, the hinges rust and refuse to move. The T'ai Chi and Qigong movements, while basically simple, do require you to think about them, at least in your beginning practice. Later, you think about your breathing, and later still, about your energy flow.

Mental Vacation

Doing your T'ai Chi exercises is like taking a daily vacation for your mind. When performing them, you forget about your troubles in the "outside" world and focus only on the present moment, a moment full of slow and graceful movement and tranquil thoughts.

Spiritual Benefits of T'ai Chi Practice

The spiritual benefits of T'ai Chi exercises are a bit more difficult to define for the typical Western practitioner. Certainly, the ability to calm down and breathe deeply helps one to achieve a more open-minded viewpoint concerning one's spirituality, and enables an internal dialogue with one's belief system.

If the spirituality of a person can be judged by how he or she treats others, then T'ai Chi can indeed develop the spirit. When you feel better and more energized, you will treat others with more compassion. The mental escape from your everyday problems may allow you to realize that your problems are actually quite insignificant, compared with the universal view of things.

A person who is at peace with himself, often referred to as an enlightened being, is also at peace with the world around him. Herein lies perhaps the ultimate goal of T'ai Chi practice.

Qi: What is it?

The Chinese word *Qi*, often spelled Chi, has several meanings ascribed to it, but for our purposes in T'ai Chi practice, it would be well to view Qi as "energy." It is seen as the prime material of life—without Qi, you are not alive. It is the driving force, the primal material, that unknowable quality that allows us to live.

Qi has been likened to adrenaline and to blood, and in some ways this may be an apt comparison. Like adrenaline, Qi can be tapped for emergency situations where great amounts of strength are required. But unlike adrenaline, we learn to bring forth this energy at will through our T'ai Chi practice, rather than waiting for the appropriate set of circumstances. Like blood, it flows through the body in a series of canals and rivers, roughly equivalent to veins and arteries.

All of Traditional Chinese Medicine practice is based on the concept of Qi (see Chapter 12), and because T'ai Chi can be viewed as a therapeutic exercise based on Chinese medicine, it follows that T'ai Chi practice involves the recognition, development, and use of Qi. This does not necessarily happen in the first days or weeks of practice—indeed, it may be years before you begin to feel this energy. Some of my students have felt the manifestation of Qi in their hands after only one or two classes, usually as a sensation of heat and/or a subtle tingling of the fingers. Others have not yet learned to recognize the feeling, even after years of lessons. Each student will have a different path in achieving the goal of energy manipulation, but in the meantime, they will benefit on the physical and mental fronts.

If you have ever had acupuncture, acupressure, Reiki, Healing Touch, or other alternative healing methods, you have perhaps unknowingly been subjected to Qi flow. It may have been your Qi, it may have been the therapist's Qi, or it may have been a combination. But these modalities all invoke this energy source through different methods to heal and strengthen the patient.

Perhaps the best way to approach this concept of Qi at this beginning stage of your T'ai Chi experience is to keep an open mind, be aware of how your body feels both before and after your T'ai Chi or Qigong practice, and don't try too hard to feel Qi. Just relax, enjoy the exercises in their own right, and someday you may be the proud owner of a fully-recognized Qi flow.

According to Chinese medical thought, Qi flows throughout every living creature. Qi moves throughout the body in little "rivers," or pathways called meridians and channels. There are 12 meridians and eight channels in the human body, as well as dozens of lesser pathways of no immediate interest to this discussion.

The T'ai Chi and Qigong movements are used to aid the Qi in its journey through these pathways, to dissolve blockages that can lead to sickness and disease, and to increase your general energy level. At higher levels of practice, you visualize this energy moving through different channels, depending on what part of your body you wish to work on. So if you want to work on your lungs, for example, you would perform certain exercises that are known to affect the Lung Meridian. In my clinical practice, when I prescribe T'ai Chi exercises to my patients, I know through my diagnosis which meridian or channel is not flowing properly, and I teach a simple movement to perform several times per day to alleviate the problem. In many of the exercises in this book, I will be describing what meridian is involved in the movement, so you will get a good idea which movements to use for which ailments— sort of like prescribing your own wellness program.

Qi has a long and distinguished history, having been recognized by Chinese physicians more than 5,000 years ago. They theorized that Qi was the common denominator in all living things, that it was the glue that connected us with the universe. Just as people are different from animals and plants, so is the energy contained within them. In ascending order, the refinement of Qi starts with minerals, then proceeds to plants, animals, humans, and the universe. Each of these five levels has its own type and amount of energy, so if you were describing the energy of a rock, for instance, you might describe it as solid, unyielding, and heavy, while the universal energy is often described as all-encompassing, light, and ethereal. It is all the same energy, it just manifests itself differently at each level.

Qi is also divided into two phases known as "yin" and "yang." It is the job of exercises such as T'ai Chi to balance these two aspects of the body's energy. We will explore the concept of yin and yang in more depth in Chapter 12.

T'ai Chi or Qigong?

"So, what is this Qigong stuff? I thought this was a book on T'ai Chi."

It is. That's why we will learn Qigong. Confused? That's okay—it gets clearer.

In Chapter 3, we will explore the history and components of Qigong (pronounced "Chee-Goong"), but for now, a few words on why you should *not* practice T'ai Chi.

You should *not* practice T'ai Chi, at least the usual forms of T'ai Chi, when you first begin exploring the Chinese healing and movement arts. Why? Because it's so confusing. Does the expression, "can't chew gum and walk at the same time" apply to you? If not, you may proceed to the later chapters where we introduce T'ai Chi movement principles.

But if you have ever wondered just how coordinated you are…if you have a fear of falling down because of a bad hip or bad legs…if you think you have poor balance…if you constantly bump into things…don't worry. You can still do T'ai Chi, but must begin at the beginning: Chapter 3. If you are confined to a sitting position, that's okay too—we'll get to T'ai Chi eventually, but we will approach it slightly differently.

If you are a fantastic ballroom dancer, then by all means proceed at will. But if you are like I once was—all thumbs with two oversized left feet—then perhaps the next chapter may help.

T'ai Chi's Little Sister

Qigong Basics

So, When Do I Start Doing T'ai Chi?

Not quite yet!

As you saw toward the end of the last chapter, I do NOT advocate jumping into T'ai Chi with both feet.

T'ai Chi can be a daunting learning experience. You need to be aware of and in control of (in most cases) two legs and two arms, one head, one back, a pair of hands, and a pair of feet. Not to mention hips, waist, neck, and eyes. That's a lot to think about. Add in the stepping patterns used in T'ai Chi, patterns that require you to walk in prescribed methods while performing certain arm and hand motions, and you may begin to despair that you will ever learn this T'ai Chi stuff. But don't worry. We'll sneak up on T'ai Chi by getting to know its little sister, Qigong.

I like to describe T'ai Chi as "Qigong with legs," a description that seems to fit nicely. Qigong is a series of movements that contains many of the T'ai Chi principles and most of the benefits of T'ai Chi practice, without the need for stepping around. You can perform Qigong standing, sitting down, even lying down. Now, if your specific problem is loss of balance, then you need T'ai Chi. We'll get to that soon enough. Right now, let's make the acquaintance of Qigong.

What is Qigong?

Qigong, literally "skill in working with your energy," actually predates T'ai Chi by thousands of years. It is, unlike the martially oriented T'ai Chi, a purely healing exercise. When you perform "Strum the Lute" in T'ai Chi, you are visualizing the destruction of your opponent's shoulder. When you do the same movement as a Qigong exercise, you can visualize the Qi flow coming down your arm, healing your arthritis.

Qigong is a series of exercises designed to loosen the joints; promote deep, relaxed breathing; and cure many medical ailments. It is thousands of years old, and comes in many different styles and flavors—everything from the Five Animal Qigong and Wild Goose Qigong (in which you portray an animal going about its day), to Medical Qigong (designed expressly for medical ailments, the forms we will be concentrating on in this book), to Spiritual Qigong (meant to increase your spirituality), to Sexual Qigong (you can guess what this one is for). Martial Qigong, yet another style of exercise, is aimed at the warrior looking to increase his or her martial arts ability.

The movements in Qigong exercises are all performed slowly and smoothly. They are not meant to be weight-lifting or Pilates-type exercises. On the contrary, they are designed to gently stretch and lengthen your muscles, ligaments, and tendons; increase your breathing capacity; loosen up and preserve your joints; and lead you to a calm, relaxed state of mind. Muscle is not usually used in Qigong exercises, rather, you feel as if you are suspended in a giant ball of cotton, with all of your resulting movements soft and slow. Emphasis is placed on correct posture and body alignment, removing stress from the joints, and learning to use the body in the most efficient manner possible. These movements can be done standing, seated, or prone—the choice is up to you.

Qigong is a way of building internal strength, sometimes described as will, faith, or constitution. In the Western world, prayer can serve the same purpose—to steel the resolve and visualize the perfect you. Qigong acts through many levels: physical, mental, and emotional. I have had many students over the years who, in the middle of a Qigong exercise, began crying or laughing. The movements, while simple, are powerful. They affect the physical body in a range-of-motion manner, lubricating the joints and strengthening the associated tendons, ligaments, and muscles. They clear and focus the mind, enabling you to concentrate and remember better, and they contribute to an increased sense of spirituality. All in all, they provide a wonderful set of benefits for very little investment in labor.

Qigong also stimulates blood flow to the brain. It contains many postures similar to "cross crawl" activities. These activities stimulate coordination between hemispheres of the cerebral cortex, and they enable balance and communication between the left and right sides of the body. This corresponds to balance and communication with the yin and yang of the inner self and to harmony with nature's cycles.

As a general rule, Qigong exercises do not involve stepping movements, but rather are performed in a relaxed stationary position. The emphasis is on proper breathing and postural alignment, as well as Qi flow. The slow speed of the motions, often described as "moving in water," lend a meditative aspect to the exercises, and allow the practitioner to focus on the physical movements to the exclusion of all outside stimuli. This single-focus technique is useful as a mini-vacation from the worries and problems of your life.

So now we'll be learning some Qigong exercises in order to practice the basic principles of T'ai Chi. It's like learning the alphabet before you can start to form words. One of the nice things about Qigong exercises is that if you are unable to stand for extended periods, or are confined to a wheelchair, it is possible to still use these exercises and enjoy their many benefits, in a manner that we will explore in Chapter 8.

Qigong's relationship with T'ai Chi is an intimate one. Both exercises utilize Qi, are mindful of proper body mechanics, and use deep breathing and relaxation techniques to produce the final fluid motions of the body. The mental outlook when performing either of these arts is similar: A quiet, focused mind is essential to gain the maximum benefit. The one main difference between the two is that T'ai Chi is a martial art, somewhat similar to Kung Fu. The T'ai Chi movements, while usually seen performed in a slow-motion manner, can be speeded up to provide a superior form of self-defense. The combination of linear and round movements, coupled with the proper flow of internal energy, gives a fighting art that is distinct and highly effective. The one drawback in all this is that it takes years to learn T'ai Chi as a self-defense system. The student needs to have a deep understanding, and a "body memory," of the T'ai Chi movements, and needs to have practiced many times with a Master to realize the full extent of this fighting art.

For those wishing to use T'ai Chi as a healing or relaxation exercise, years of study are not required. With a good teacher, the typical student can begin to learn the fundamental movements of T'ai Chi within a week. Granted, it may take a bit longer to master the full form, but within a reasonable length of time, you can be practicing the form on your own. My students typically come to me for a year or so, learn the form and all of the attendant variations and subtleties, and then go off and practice on their own. They may start the learning process by coming to class two or three times per week, but when they have the form "internalized," they come only once a week or so, to refresh and refine their art.

The overall effect from Qigong training is gained through persistent and dedicated practice over months and years. Because there are so many methods out there, it is generally advisable to pick one type to start with, and to gain the benefits that are promised from its practice, before moving on to another more complicated method. You should also know that it is inadvisable to train in two types of Qigong that are not congruent with one another, that is to say, do not mix hard and soft Qigong methods. When you train in Qigong, you are making changes to your energetic system and also your endocrine system.

With the Qigong instruction contained in this book, I can guarantee you that after only one hour of trying the movements, you will have exercises that you will remember and can practice at any time.

Styles and Types of Qigong

Although there are thousands of Qigong exercises available, they all can be classified into one of five main schools, or styles, of Qigong. This is not to say that a certain exercise cannot be used for both medical and spiritual purposes, for example, but as a general tool of convenience and as a learning aid, the following five styles will be explored in this section:

1. **The Taoist school** stresses the preservation of the physical body. The Taoist styles emphasize joint health, internal and external strength-building, balance, deep breathing, and relaxation.

2. **The Buddhist school** is aimed at liberating the mind through the Qigong exercises. Many Buddhist exercises are inwardly oriented to focus your attention on the spiritual aspects of your life. As a result, these are often described as static, or non-moving, Qigong exercises.

3. **The Confucian school** dwells on attaining higher moral character. Confucian Qigong has not, to this point, been utilized extensively in the United States, but is still practiced in China.

4. **The Medical school** teaches patients how to take control of their own illnesses, and also how to prevent them. The emphasis is hygienic in nature. It also teaches medical people how to use the inner Qi in a dynamic way for healing the aches and pains of others. This is the style of Qigong that we will focus on in this book.

5. **The Martial school** of Qigong focuses on protecting the body from sword cuts, blunt trauma from other-than-edged weapons, and safety from attack by fist or foot. Such methods include Iron Shirt and Golden Bell-type methods. It also trains the body to deliver fatal blows that are enhanced with Qi, such as those found in Burning Palm or Iron Palm methods.

Within the various schools of Qigong, you will find very simple and easy-to-do sets, such as the 18-Movement Qigong and Eight Pieces of Brocade, to more complicated methods such as Wild Goose Qigong and Falun Gong. All have their relative merits and drawbacks, so once you progress to the stage where you are looking for a new Qigong form, choose carefully.

Now let's examine Medical Qigong a bit more closely, as the exercises in this book are taken from that school.

Introduction to Medical Qigong

Traditional Chinese Medicine (TCM) is a holistic system for promoting health through the use of several therapies such as acupuncture, herbal medicine, acupressure massage, and Medical Qigong. These therapies are often used in various combinations.

The central theory of TCM is to balance the Qi (the vital energy in the body) according to several theories such as Yin-Yang, Five Element, and Six Stages. These theories are used in TCM in general as well as in Medical Qigong in particular.

In the **Yin-Yang Theory**, all of life is composed of two opposing yet complementary forces: the yin (feminine, dark, weak) and the yang (masculine, light, strong). At birth, the human body normally contains equal amounts of both traits. When sickness develops, it can be attributed to a deficiency or excess of either of the two forces. Medical Qigong seeks to restore this balance through movement and breathing exercises.

The **Five Element Theory** states that all things in the universe, including humans, have a collection of traits that correspond to five natural Elements: Wood, Fire, Metal, Earth, and Water. Within each of these elements is found a certain physical and mental representation:

Wood: Liver, growth at birth, yang.

Fire: Heart, maximum growth, yang.

Metal: Lungs, declining functions, yin.

Earth: Spleen, stabilization, balanced between yin and yang.

Water: Kidneys, rest, yin.

Qigong exercises affect the actions of the five Elements in the body through Qi flow. Thus, a person who is diagnosed as being Water deficient may have exercises prescribed to improve that Element, thus aiding kidney function. An expert in Medical Qigong is often also a Chinese medicine practitioner, as the ability to diagnose the five Element signs is vital to both fields.

The **Six Stages Theory** uses the idea that disease attacks certain organs and organ systems according to severity and level of infection. For example, the "Great Yang Stage" sickness affects the exterior of the body, in addition to the small intestine and bladder, while the "Terminal Yin Stage" affects the pericardium and liver organs and strikes deep within the body. According to the proper diagnosis using this theory, exercises would again be prescribed to alleviate the disease.

A more detailed account of Traditional Chinese Medicine can be found in Chapter 12.

So, how exactly does all of this affect you? The exercises that you will learn here are designed to give your body a "tune up" at many different levels. They have been refined and tested over thousands of years specifically with medical concerns in mind. So when you do the exercises in their proper form and sequence, you will be stimulating the meridians and channels in the body to enhance the flow of healthy energy (Qi) while at the same time eliminating the unhealthy energy (Sha Qi). Because of the positions assumed during the movements, you are alternately compressing and expanding the energy rivers, in addition to exercising the muscles, tendons, ligaments, and joints. By learning proper posture and diaphragmatic breathing, you are aiding your body in maintaining optimal health and fitness. The twisting of the waist and hips, along with the spinal stimulation, helps to massage the internal organs and the tissue surrounding them. While all of this activity is taking place, you are maintaining a calm and relaxed mental state through your focus on the simple movements. Thus you are taking a break from your worries and sicknesses through the practice of Medical Qigong.

Precautions

The exercises contained and taught in this book are designed to be easy to learn for the general population, but there can be times when a particular movement causes undue pain or discomfort. When this happens, STOP. Don't keep pressing on in hopes that the pain will subside, or because you have to "tough it out."

T'ai Chi and Qigong are exercises that are supposed to be relaxing while being energetically stimulating. Students often comment on how much more "alive" they feel after their practice. So why should you experience pain? One reason may be that you are performing the movement incorrectly. Often, the simple re-adjustment of a shoulder or wrist can be the difference between relaxation and stress, so you might like to review the instructions and photos, and determine if this is the cause of your problem.

Another possibility is that your medical condition simply does not allow the movement to be performed. In advanced cases of arthritis and carpal tunnel syndrome, every movement can feel like a fire burning in your joints. In a case such as this, once again, STOP. Think about where the pain is located, if it is a "flare-up" or a low-key type of pain. Have you experienced this pain prior to doing the exercises? If so, take a rest for a while. Then come back and try the exercise again, this time slowing the movement down and decreasing the size of the motions. If an exercise requires you to lift your arms over your head, and that is the point at which the pain begins, modify the movement so that the arms only come up halfway.

There is no hard and fast rule concerning Qigong, other than that you should enjoy it. Don't feel like you are "cheating" or not getting any benefit by going halfway. Remember, "If there's pain, you're not using your brain."

Finally, there are some practitioners who simply cannot stand up in one place long enough to complete the exercises. For these students, I have devoted a separate chapter to seated adaptations of Qigong and T'ai Chi (see Chapter 8). It is true that you won't be able to work on your balance problems while seated, but let's take it one step at a time, shall we? Get the blood and Qi moving, and focus on your breathing while you do the seated exercises. Many of the benefits of these movements are aimed at the upper body, so you will lose little by practicing seated forms.

Remember also not to fixate on perfect form. Often in my classes and demonstrations, a person will comment, "I could never be that graceful," or "Oh, he makes it look so easy, but I'm a complete klutz." Wrong. The goal is not to look like Fred and Ginger, but to get healthy. Some people have a native elegance to their movements, an elegance that seems to have run out by the time you got to the supply window. Don't worry! Work on the movements without thinking how it looks. Many students will comment, "I don't want anyone watching me—I feel so silly." Rubbish. No one is looking at you—they're all trying to figure out how to do their *own* movements!

In time, with conscientious practice, you will discover that you are suddenly moving in a more graceful manner, that your body seems to work more efficiently, and that you can go for longer periods without tiring. That's the true magic of these movements.

Remember that one of the benefits of doing T'ai Chi is that you learn to relax your body, to feel comfortable within yourself, and to move in a whole new way— a relaxed and graceful way. Fighting the movements when you are learning will only become counterproductive: You will strive and try your hardest, but the movement will seem to recede faster and faster, until you get discouraged and quit altogether. Then you will never gain the benefits that millions of others have.

A note here for students with physical disabilities such as being confined to a wheelchair, or those with fibromyalgia or arthritis who cannot stand for long periods of time. Again, do what you can in a comfortable manner, and if you start to feel pain, stop immediately. Don't push it beyond your limits. Remember that you can adapt every one of these movements to your own particular circumstances.

As always, it is a good idea to check with your doctor before you begin any exercise program. While T'ai Chi is probably the least strenuous exercise that you could practice, it's still vital to know your state of physical ability. In more than 30 years of practice, I have encountered two cases in which a student was advised not to practice T'ai Chi. The first was a kidney-transplant recipient, fresh out of the hospital. It is understandable that there was a necessary recuperation period after such an operation. The other instance was when the student's doctor did not understand what T'ai Chi was, believing it to be, in his own words, "jumping around like a maniac and getting all sweated up."

Not being one to let the good name of T'ai Chi be dragged down, I promptly arranged a visit to that doctor, where I proceeded to demonstrate the exercises involved. The doctor had thought T'ai Chi was a kissing cousin of Karate, and had visions of his patient in white pajamas, breaking boards and screaming like a maniac. The good doctor learned about T'ai Chi that day, and I gained a long-time student.

But do listen to your doctor's advice, and if he or she is not familiar with T'ai Chi (an increasingly rare occurrence), then offer to bring in some printed materials or arrange to have the T'ai Chi teacher contact the doctor. You'll be doing yourself, and T'ai Chi, a world of good.

Chapter 4

On Your Mark, Get Set, Relax!

Preparing for T'ai Chi Play

Physical Settings for T'ai Chi

While it is true that you could theoretically practice T'ai Chi anywhere, there are certain locations that lend themselves better than others. Considerations such as amount of space, noise, temperature and humidity levels, and number of distractions in the form of people and animals should be included in your choice of practice area.

The amount of space needed to practice T'ai Chi varies with the style and specific form that you are practicing. A Chen Style form using an 8-foot staff would certainly require much more space than the Eight Pieces of Brocade Qigong (see Chapter 6 for more information on this Qigong form). The T'ai Chi and Qigong exercises in this book are designed to take up the minimum of space—as little as the distance between your outstretched hands. This is not to suggest you practice in your walk-in closet! There are other considerations you'll need to think about.

For a basic T'ai Chi moving form, such as the Yang Style 24-Movement Form, your space needs will increase only slightly—perhaps a 10-x-12-foot space would be sufficient. Of course, the more space the better, so if you are blessed with a really large living room, or have a nice little backyard, then you've probably found your perfect practice area.

Outdoor Practice Areas

Speaking of backyards, what about practicing outdoors? Well, certainly your location, as well as the season and daily weather, will be primary considerations. In Northeast Pennsylvania, where I am, we seem to have two seasons: winter and summer. Somewhere along the way, we lost fall and spring. As a result of this meteorological oddity, we usually cannot go outside to practice until sometime in late April, and begin to move back indoors in September. Of course, during the midsummer heat waves, we elect to stay in our air-conditioned studio. Remember: If there's pain, you're not using your brain! If you are lucky enough to reside in states with more moderate climates, such as California or Florida, then the changing seasons are not as big a consideration.

With these facts in mind, let's explore a few choice locations for T'ai Chi play, starting with outdoor locations.

Parks

In nice weather, parks are wonderful for T'ai Chi practice. The communion with nature, the singing birds, the slight warm breeze, perhaps the sound of water flowing in a stream, all help to calm you down and add another dimension to your practice. The ground is soft under your feet, the sun is shining, and everything is right with the world.

Until the kids' softball team comes out to practice. Then you might have problems. In a public park, you are at the mercy of a space used by other members of the public using the space at the same time you are. The youthful shouts of glee may gladden the heart, but do nothing for your concentration and focus. Add to that the folks who are out for a nice stroll who stop to watch you practice. Now, this doesn't bother me, because I'm a bit of a show-off and know that I'm good at what I do, but if you are the least bit unsure of your ability, or are a little shy around strangers, then the park might not be the best place for you. Remember, there's a balance in all things—you'll have advantages and drawbacks at every location you choose.

Rural Locations

If you are lucky enough to have some woods nearby, or a nice desolate little meadow, then take advantage of it. You'll have all the advantages of the park with none of the drawbacks. Or will you…?

I once found what I thought was a perfect location for my daily practice while I was traveling through New Hampshire. It was a thickly wooded area, tall majestic trees towering overhead, and a lush carpet of grass underneath. The sun was shining and the birds were singing. I settled myself, meditated for a few minutes, and began my exercises.

At first, it was just a little itch on the side of my neck, not enough to distract me from my practice. Then another itch, and another, then a bite, then two bites. I was being introduced to the notorious fly population of the area. Soon, a swarm was forming around me, and all thoughts of T'ai Chi were abandoned as I ran to find shelter indoors. So much for the big, bad T'ai Chi teacher!

Flies notwithstanding, a rural location has much to offer the T'ai Chi practitioner.

Beach/Lake/Stream/River

Ah, water, the essence of life; the universal solvent.

Water is highly symbolic in T'ai Chi and Qigong. In your practice, you are attempting to imitate the qualities of water—strong yet yielding, always flowing, assuming the shape of whatever container (or area) you find yourself in. Through its constant flowing, water, as soft as it is, can wear down the largest boulder in the stream. In colder climes, water can split open rocks by entering fissures and then freezing. Water can also change into the gaseous state of steam, showing yet another side of its abilities.

So, in our practice, we seek to emulate water for both its gentle flowing ability and its strength under pressure. Practicing T'ai Chi in the immediate vicinity of water can do much for the visualization of these characteristics. In addition, the sound of the water, whether in a bubbling stream or as crashing surf, has a relaxing effect on many people. My personal preference is to practice at the ocean on the beach. The soft sand underfoot, the gulls all around, the smell and sound of the water's eternal movement, all relax me and connect me to the primal qualities of water in my exercises.

Athletic Fields

If you have a school or college near you, you might be able to use the athletic field as a practice site. The advantages are that you have virtually unlimited space, and if there is not a practice going on, you'll usually also have peace and quiet.

The sole disadvantage is that, with all of today's security considerations, athletic fields are sometimes locked up during down times, and you might need to be a member of the school or college to utilize the field. But it's certainly worth the effort to investigate your area and find out if this big practice area is available to you.

Your Yard

Home Sweet Home! Why bother to walk or drive to the park or field if you are lucky enough to have a yard at your home or apartment complex. The main advantage is, of course, location, because you can be close to home and yet have the benefits of outdoor practice. You are familiar with the territory, setting your mind at ease, and are unlikely to be bothered by gawkers.

That being said, if your yard is in front of your home and borders on a public thoroughfare, be ready for some odd looks and occasional questions from passersby. Depending on your mood, you may wish to take a break from your practice to socialize with your newfound friends, or you may simply wish to ignore them. Better, if at all possible, is to practice in a yard shielded from the street, either by location (a backyard is ideal), a deck in the back of the house (or a balcony in your apartment), or by using a fence to block the view of the curious.

I've had several students over the years get so involved in their T'ai Chi practice that they created little sanctuaries in their backyards, complete with landscaping, waterfalls, and ponds. One student even had hidden outdoor speakers installed so that he could play relaxing music while practicing outside. Another commissioned a large entranceway to his backyard practice area in the form of a large Chinese gateway, complete with carved dragons and phoenixes. Now you don't need to go to those lengths to enjoy your T'ai Chi—just clear out the grandchildren's toys and devote a small area for yourself.

Indoor Practice Areas

Now to the indoor locations. Indoor practice has the advantage of shelter from weather and pests, is usually available on a scheduled basis, and is generally less distracting than outdoor practice. Certainly, climate control is often the most-quoted advantage of working indoors, and I agree. It's nice not to be perspiring or freezing when you practice, or batting at the flies and mosquitoes that think you're dinner.

Here are five indoor locations for your consideration.

Your Home or Apartment

If you have or can make the space, whether on a temporary or permanent basis, you would be wise to consider this option first. It costs nothing extra (except perhaps a few minutes of time to move that magazine rack out of your way) and is the ultimate in convenience. If you wake up at 3 a.m. and want to practice, your space is ready. You also have access to bathroom facilities, water, and music, if you choose.

Your T'ai Chi School

I would be remiss if I didn't mention this one! A school devoted solely to T'ai Chi may not be in your immediate neighborhood, and you might not wish to attend one even if it were. Shyness, apprehension, and fear of being seen as a "beginner" all contribute to some people's reluctance to attend a public T'ai Chi school.

But if you give it a chance, you may wonder why you didn't do this years ago. The school usually has a small number of students practicing at any one time, so you shouldn't worry about overcrowding unless the school is extremely small. You will probably be together with like-minded individuals with whom you will often establish a bond of friendship, often extending outside of the school. The decor may put you in a relaxed, meditative state of mind, furthering the effectiveness of your practice.

In my main school in Kingston, Pennsylvania, I have gone to some lengths to create a comfortable atmosphere for my students. Everything from the lighting (overhead recessed flood lights controlled by dimmer switches), the paint on the walls (muted colors in a marble pattern, chosen to produce a relaxed frame of mind), the miniature indoor waterfall, and the little collectibles and display items (all related in some way to Chinese culture) is designed to produce a tranquil state of mind, and to ensure that the student's time here is happy and productive. The imported sandalwood incense is burning and the music is softly playing; all contribute to a meditative atmosphere.

This isn't to say that the T'ai Chi school in your area will be the same—some have just a bare room with painted-over windows, no air-conditioning, no music, and lots of noise from neighboring businesses. But if you learn the basics of T'ai Chi, it won't matter, because you'll be traveling on your inner journey.

Community Center

A community center can be a great choice for T'ai Chi practice. The camaraderie you can experience there is wonderful and can add immeasurably to your practice sessions. Often, a community center will offer a four- or six-week course in T'ai Chi, so you could have your instruction and practice it, too.

Senior Center

Senior centers are spread all over the land, and usually offer several advantages for the T'ai Chi player. You could practice among your peers and make lots of new friends. Also, senior centers rarely charge for use of the space, and there are other activities you can partake of both before and after your T'ai Chi practice. You might even get a little group going, and end up being a T'ai Chi teacher!

Hospitals/Rehabilitation Centers

Hospitals and rehab centers are increasingly growing aware of the benefits of T'ai Chi, and usually have either classes available or a space in which you can practice. If your doctor tells you that T'ai Chi would be a good exercise for you, perhaps he or she could arrange for the use of some space at these locations on a weekly basis—an unused conference room or therapy area would be ideal.

Choosing an Instructor and a School

Finding a school and an instructor is not an easy task. In my case, I studied with two teachers for 25 years (total). From one teacher, I did not learn much; to the other, I owe my life in T'ai Chi. Although what I learned was valuable and enticing, I knew there must be more. They both knew a lot, but one of them did not teach the way I expected—pretty much on purpose. This was in New York's Chinatown in the 1970s. There were two classes of teachers: older Chinese who "knew something," and hippies who thought they knew T'ai Chi, but really knew very few of the details. The one who changed my life, an elderly Chinese gentleman, was the one who taught in an unorthodox manner.

There are at least two factors about T'ai Chi that would set up a circumstance such as the situation I describe above.

The first is that much of what goes on in T'ai Chi is internal; it is called an internal martial art for good reason. The external movement, unless you already know much, is deceiving, because all the activity is hidden inside the body. My favorite example is that when people watch T'ai Chi, they think the arms are moving. Generally, however, the arms aren't moving (though they look as if they are); what is really happening is that the body is moving the arms. This phenomenon of moving the arms by the body does cause the arms to move through space, but only as an unmoving appendage to the body and not separately from the body the way we generally move our arms in everyday life, that is, independently from the body.

So, the job of the teacher is to convey this training, level upon level, as the student is able to grasp and implement the information and integrate the skills into his or her own body.

The second factor is that in the Orient, much of this knowledge is rightly considered valuable, and traditionally has been hidden. So there is a tradition of not speaking plainly about what is going on inside the body and actually withholding instruction. How you achieved becoming instructed traditionally was complex and usually involved "proving yourself" and forming a close personal relationship with your teacher, earning his trust and good will until he was willing to show you what was really going on inside the body.

You can view it this way: There is an inner circle and an outer circle. The inner circle is like family where instruction is given eagerly; the outer circle is where more "outside" knowledge is transmitted without much explanation. In the first two years of my T'ai Chi training, I was in the outer circle, aware that there was more to learn. I finally found a teacher who knew the art and was willing to teach me the inner circle. To him, I am eternally grateful.

Things are different now in the 21st century. There are a number of Westerners who have received good instruction on the internal aspects of T'ai Chi and are willing to teach. There are more Asians with good training who are willing to teach the internal aspects. There is no rating system for T'ai Chi teachers, though, such as the black belt system. The art is also immense, with many aspects and many styles that emphasize different aspects of the art. There are commonalties between the styles, but also different emphases, so going between one style and another can be confusing (at least in the beginning of your training).

What you want in the beginning of your training is to build a good foundation in T'ai Chi, to learn the fundamentals well. Then you can sample differences and integrate them into your foundation as a refinement, but only once the basics have been learned.

So you want a teacher with good knowledge, who has received good instruction. Ask him about his training. How many years did he train? Did he study other styles of martial arts at the same time? If so, his views of T'ai Chi may be slightly influenced by those styles. You can find a good teacher with only five or so years of training, but it certainly helps to have more. Ask him what he has learned. Can he demonstrate his answers with movements? Ask about what goes on inside the Form—the breathing techniques, the energy flows—and how these things all provide benefits.

Ask about Qigong and what his experience has been with Qigong. As we discussed earlier, Qigong is the art of breathing and energy flow, which has been incorporated into T'ai Chi. It is one of the major transformative aspects of the art and also one of the most important aspects for improving and maintaining health. Breath-work is often not incorporated into the Form in the beginning of training, but you want an instructor who has knowledge of it. The breath is ultimately the heart of T'ai Chi and you will want to know how to integrate Qigong breathing into your T'ai Chi. Obviously, if you are in a rural area, it may be difficult to find a very experienced instructor and you will study with whoever is available. But you should keep in mind that there are very high levels of instruction available in the United States and around the world today, and, ultimately, you may want to partake in this instruction as your abilities grow. There are many fine workshops given throughout the year in many areas of the country that you can attend and receive great instruction. There are regular listings in T'ai Chi magazines and Websites. Two magazines that immediately come to mind are *T'ai Chi* magazine and *Qi—The*

Journal of Chinese Health. A few good Internet sites are the Tai Chi Message Board (*http://gate8.com/bbs-tai/messages/tai-chi34.html*), which offers a message board of questions about T'ai Chi, including announcements of workshops; and the Taijiquan Club (*www.annualfestival@taijiquanclub.com/*), which offers a calendar of workshops around the world. You do, however, want to find an instructor in your area from whom you can learn on a weekly basis.

In my experience, there are three levels of instruction: teaching, coaching, and training. You need all three to learn good T'ai Chi.

Teaching is where things are explained to an entire class at one time, and each person goes off alone or works with others (in the case of push-hands) to incorporate the instructions into their form, their bodies, and the art.

Coaching is where the instructor works with you individually, giving you something to practice during the week, instructions on how to do it and what it will feel like. You will report back the following week how it felt and demonstrate what you learned.

Training is where the instructor works with you, gives you forms to try, and asks you what it feels like. If you are doing it incorrectly, he will give you something else to try or show you how to correct what is wrong while telling you how it should feel. Each time, the instructor looks for improvement until you get it right. You practice at home and continue to build on what you learn each week.

When I teach, it is individual instruction in a group setting. There is some general instruction, but I get around to each person in every class to take him or her to the next step in his or her training. Each person hears differently, has a different body, and needs to be dealt with individually as they learn. Obviously, my private classes are small—not usually more than 12 people. Public classes can exceed 50 people in a class. The classes at my school run an hour long, and we work on stretching, fundamental training exercises, form instruction, and meditation. Keep in mind, this is not the only way to teach. In a lot of larger schools, people learn as a group with junior instructors until they gain enough fundamental knowledge to benefit from individual work with the founder of the school. Both have their benefits.

The personality of the instructor is also important. The transmission of T'ai Chi is from teacher to student and is a fairly intimate activity. It is similar to raising a child or being raised by a parent. You need your own boundaries as a person and you need to distinguish between what is T'ai Chi and what is the personality of the teacher—in the transmission of T'ai Chi they often get mixed together (this is one reason for the different T'ai Chi styles). So, it is important that you are able to accept the personality of the teacher, even though you might not see the world in the same way he or she does. You will be absorbing the teacher's influence, so it is important to pay attention to who he or she is as a person and keep distinguishing the teacher as separate from the art being taught or the philosophy of the teacher. There may be some personalities from which you will choose not to learn.

As I write this, it occurs to me that all this seems like a lot to take on. And it *is* a lot to take on. It is really worth it, though. T'ai Chi is incredibly rich, magical, healthy, powerful, and fulfilling. I look on it as one of the great gifts to the people of this planet; without its existence, we would be much poorer. To me, it is like the medicinal plants in the rain forest—full of hidden treasure and value from which we can learn so much to enrich our lives and health.

Time of Day to Practice

Chinese wisdom holds that the hours of the day are divided into two separate times: the energizing hours and the relaxing hours. This division has much to do with Traditional Chinese Medicine, which says that your Qi is more active in certain body areas at certain times than at others. Even the quality of the energy varies according to the time of day, so it might be important to take these facts into account in planning your T'ai Chi practice times.

Generally, the morning hours are devoted to energizing the body, in preparation for the day's activities. So when you practice your T'ai Chi early in the morning, you are greeting the day and gathering up and focusing your energy and your spirit. This is why millions of Chinese T'ai Chi players exercise at the break of dawn in their public parks—they know that they are attuning themselves to a universal energy source by practicing at those times. It just seems to make your whole day go better, with more energy and less conflict, when you do your T'ai Chi in the morning.

Evenings, on the other hand, should be for relaxing. The same T'ai Chi exercises, done with a different mindset, can be performed in the evenings for slowing down and readying for sleep. Indeed, T'ai Chi has often had this effect on my students—they become so relaxed, they almost fall asleep while exercising.

One thing to watch out for, though, is when your evening practice seems to energize instead of relax you. I have had a number of students who simply cannot practice T'ai Chi after 6 p.m., because it gives them so much energy that they are up all night, scurrying around the house and cleaning everything in sight! You'll know, after your first few practice sessions, whether this applies to you.

Core Concepts of T'ai Chi: Breathing, Alignment, Energy

Here's where we finally start to look at the basic principles of Qigong and T'ai Chi exercises. These principles are perhaps the most important phase of learning these arts, so please go slowly and learn them well. Don't gloss over them just because they seem boring or obvious—within these principles is the *real* magic of T'ai Chi.

Breathing

Breathing is the soul of T'ai Chi—without proper breathing, you'll never gain all of the benefits possible, and will just be performing a dance. True, that dance will help loosen and strengthen your joints, but the internal healing that can occur will be absent.

The preferred method of breathing in T'ai Chi is called diaphragmatic breathing. It uses the diaphragm, a sheet of muscle located below your lungs, to pull air into and push air out of your lungs in the most efficient manner possible. Most people are what I call "top breathers"—they breathe shallowly, using only the top-third portion of their lungs, and never reach their full capacity. This acts to restrict the amount of oxygen the bloodstream can receive, thus starving your body for food.

By using the diaphragm, you will pull air into the very bottom portions of your lungs and reap the benefits accordingly. You'll have more energy, you'll breathe easier, and your health will vastly improve.

So, what is this diaphragmatic breathing technique? It's really quite simple. Place one hand on your lower abdomen, just below your navel. Now place the other hand on your chest at heart level. You will be breathing through your nose for these exercises, so if you have asthma or a deviated septum, modify accordingly. But *do* try to inhale and exhale through the nostrils.

Now, inhale. As you do so, imagine that you just ate a big meal, and your stomach is expanding. Make believe that air is being pulled down into your lower abdomen (which is physically impossible, of course, unless you have some leaky plumbing). Feel your lower hand start to push out as your abdomen swells slightly. Then imagine, still on the inhale, that the lungs are filling up with air, that you can feel it pouring into all spaces in the lungs. The hand on your chest is now rising slightly. You are a balloon being inflated.

Now for the exhale. Once again, the lower hand will move first. As you begin your exhale, contract your lower abdominal muscles so that you get a "flat tummy." This will force the diaphragm upward, pushing air out of the lungs. Follow the abdominal contraction with a slight "caving in" of the chest, forcing the rest of the air out of the lungs. Congratulations—you are breathing diaphragmatically!

Of course, this all takes practice. So much so that I would advise that you only practice this breathing technique by itself for the first few weeks. Don't worry about incorporating it into your T'ai Chi yet—just practice it by itself, perhaps as you lie down in bed before going to sleep. Take five minutes and practice it every night, and before you know it, you'll be breathing to a whole new tune!

Alignment

Body alignment, or "body mechanics" as I sometimes call it, is a vital part of T'ai Chi. So many of us have spent our lives with poor posture, despite Mom's constant reminders to "sit up straight" and "don't slouch," that we don't recognize good posture when we see (or feel) it. But without the right alignment, your breathing and energy flow will suffer.

Let's start with the standing position used throughout T'ai Chi and Qigong exercises. Often referred to as Neutral Position, it is designed to be efficient and relaxed, to enable you to perform your exercises in the easiest possible fashion. Place your feet parallel to each other, pointing straight ahead, about shoulder-width apart. Let your knees bend slightly—not so much that you look like Groucho Marx, but just a little, so that they're not locked. Let the pelvis tilt slightly forward and upward, that is, tuck in your bottom, so that the bottom curvature of your spine is not so pronounced. This also, on a higher level of practice, opens the energy pathways for your Qi to flow.

Your head should be upright, not stiff-necked, but as if an invisible string is pulling upwards from the crown of your head. This will further serve to lengthen and straighten your spine. Your gaze is level and relaxed; your chin tucked in just slightly. Finally, the areas that often hold the most stress—your shoulders and arms—should hang comfortably at your sides. When you have achieved all of this positioning, you are now in Neutral Position. It may feel uncomfortable at first, and your legs and back may get tired after a few minutes, but keep practicing— over time, it will become a natural position. When we age, our spine often starts to curl forward and our legs get weak. This contributes to many of the falls that seniors experience. But if you maintain a Neutral Position in your everyday life, you'll soon find that your balance has improved greatly, that you breathe easier, and that your movements are more flowing and graceful. People will comment on your newfound appearance, and that will urge you to practice even more.

Energy

Energy, or Qi as we call it here, is the substance that makes T'ai Chi what it is: a healing art. By assuming the proper body alignment and practicing diaphragmatic breathing, we open up the rivers in which Qi flows. By doing this, the Qi can access all parts of our bodies and heal both internal and external sickness. We move our bodies as we do in T'ai Chi to stimulate and guide this energy flow.

Qi is seen in Chinese philosophy, medicine, and martial arts as being the substance of life, the spark that keeps us going. Along with blood, it travels throughout the body through multiple pathways, acting as a guardian against sickness and as a source of health and strength. We will examine the deeper qualities of Qi in Chapter 12, but for now let us invent a useful fiction that this Qi is an actual, living force in our bodies, and that by learning to recognize and control it, we can control our own health.

Part II

Living in the Present

Chapter 5

Dem Bones, Dem Bones, Dem Cold Bones

Warm-Up Exercises

Why Do Warm-Ups?

Although it is true that T'ai Chi and Qigong serve as their own warm-ups, it is still often a good practice to perform some gentle warm-ups before starting your exercises. Just as you stretch after you wake up in the morning, so too should you stretch and take a few breaths before starting the T'ai Chi exercises.

The following stretches are designed to be performed in a loose, relaxed fashion—no hard pulling or pushing, no straining to get that last inch of stretch in the muscles. Follow the basic principles of T'ai Chi play: no undue effort. As we discovered in Chapter 4, this includes keeping the elbows bent, the shoulders relaxed, the head upright, knees slightly bent, and the pelvis tilted slightly forward and upward. Even the fingers should be curled slightly, indicating a relaxed state of mind.

Warm-ups have the effect of getting the blood circulating, eliminating some of the kinks in the muscles, increasing the body temperature, and loosening up the joints. All of these points are important for the subsequent T'ai Chi movements, so do take time to perform these warm-up movements before every T'ai Chi session.

The Basic Warm-Ups

Eye Crunches

Eye warm-ups are designed to alleviate the pressure of headaches and stress that are often carried in the eyes and eye sockets (orbits). Perform these gently, without strain.

Standing or sitting comfortably, close both eyes and squeeze them tightly for five seconds, then release. Repeat five times, making sure to breathe deeply and slowly through this and all of the other warm-ups.

Now, open both eyes as wide as possible and hold for five seconds, then release. Repeat five times.

Roll both eyes to your right side, as if there is something there that you want to see, but keep your head facing forward. Bring your focus to the front and center again. Repeat five times, and then repeat on the left side five times.

Finally, roll both eyes up as far as you comfortably can, hold for five seconds, then return to center. Repeat five times. Then roll the eyes downward, as if trying to look at your feet, hold for five seconds, and return to center. Repeat five times.

Neck Bends

Contrary to popular belief, neck rolls are not good for you—in fact, they present a danger. The practice of rolling the head around on your neck in a circular motion can lead to dizziness and, more importantly, damage to the upper vertebrae. We will warm-up our necks by performing neck bends, rather than neck rolls.

With your body once again in a comfortable position, let your head tilt to the right side of your body, as if trying to touch your right shoulder with your ear. Don't force it; rather, let the weight of your head gently pull over to the side. Hold this position, while continuing to breathe, for five seconds, and then return your head to the center position. Repeat five times to the left side.

Now we will let the head tilt forward gently, again letting the weight of the head pull it forward without straining. Hold for five seconds, return to center, repeat five times. Finally, let the head tilt backward, as if looking at the ceiling, and hold for five seconds. Return to center and repeat five times.

Shoulder Shrugs

Lift both shoulders toward your ears. Hold for five seconds, remembering to breathe as you do so, then release. Repeat five times. This exercise warms the shoulder joints and loosens it up for T'ai Chi movement.

Fingers

Hold your left thumb with your fisted right hand, as if getting ready to pull your thumb outward. Pull gently, being especially careful if you have arthritis or carpal tunnel syndrome. Pull for five seconds, and then release. Repeat for each finger of the left hand.

Repeat this exercise for the right hand, using the fisted left hand to pull each finger gently for five seconds.

Now, make a tight fist with your left hand, hold for five seconds, and then release. Repeat with the right hand.

Wrists

Roll both wrists simultaneously, first in a clockwise direction, then in a counter-clockwise direction. Start with the fingers open, and perform 10 slow rolls in each direction. Then make fists of your two hands and repeat the exercise, performing 10 rolls in each direction.

Now, hold your left hand parallel to the floor in front of you, with the fingers pointing across your body to the right, at chest level. Place the palm of your right hand across the back of the left-hand fingers, and keeping the left arm horizontal, attempt to bend the left wrist downward by pressing on the left fingers. Hold for five seconds, and then release. Repeat five times. Return to the starting position.

Now place your right fingers beneath the left fingers, and press the left hand backward, as if trying to touch the back of your left forearm. Press only enough to get a good stretch—there should be no pain encountered when you perform this movement. Hold for five seconds, and then release. Repeat five times.

Now repeat both of these exercises on the right hand, making sure to breathe deeply and keep your body aligned properly.

Elbows and Shoulders

Make a loose fist with your left hand. Bring the arm across your body to the right at chest level, lifting the left elbow until it is parallel to the floor. This will look like you're trying to hug yourself with one arm, except that the elbow is raised slightly. Hold the stretch for five seconds, then release. Repeat with the right elbow.

Now back to the left side. Make a loose fist. Try to touch that fist to your left shoulder, and lift your left elbow upward toward the ceiling. Hold for five seconds, then release. Repeat with the right elbow.

Finally, with the left hand again held in a loose fist, drive the left elbow backwards, as if trying to push a wall behind you with your elbow. Keep your left fist close to the left side of the body, near your lower ribs. Hold the stretch for five seconds, and then return to the starting position. Repeat five times. Repeat on the right side.

Shoulder Circles

Start with the right arm. With the fingers open and loose, start to make circles on the right side of your body, making them as large as you comfortably can. Keep the elbow bent at all times, and breathe deeply. Make five circles with the right arm, then stop and repeat with the left arm.

Shoulder Stretches

From either a standing or seated position, reach both arms forward as far as possible, locking the elbows and straightening the fingers. You should feel as if someone is pulling your arms forward. Stretch and hold for five seconds, then relax your arms, allowing the elbows and fingers to bend slightly. Repeat five times.

For the next movement, repeat the above exercise, but with the arms stretched out to the sides instead of forward. Repeat five times.

Finally, repeat the above movements with the arms at the sides, fingers pointing toward the floor. Repeat five times.

Waist and Hips

From either a standing or seated position, be sure that your body alignment is proper—head up, feet flat, level gaze. If standing, let your arms hang at your sides; if sitting, place your hands on your knees. Bend your torso to the right side slowly, letting the weight of your upper body provide the pulling force. Breathe throughout the entire movement. Hold the stretch for five seconds and then slowly return to an upright position. Repeat five times on the left side.

Washing Machine

This is a popular warm-up that my students love. From a standing position, and keeping the feet firmly planted, slowly start to rotate your waist from side to side, allowing your relaxed arms to swing gently back and forth from left to right, then back again. You are trying to imitate the back-and-forth agitation of a washing machine—the turning of the drum is the movement you're shooting for here. Remember to keep the arms relaxed, though—no stiffness allowed. Repeat for as long as it is comfortable, combining the movements with deep, relaxed breathing. This is a wonderful warm-up for the hips, waist, and lower back.

Waist Bends

Standing upright, lock your knees so that your legs are totally straight. Inhale, and then bend forward slowly, exhaling as you do so. Let your arms dangle down in front of you as if you are trying to touch your toes. Don't force the movement—again, just let the weight of the upper body provide the pulling force.

Ankle Circles

Sit on a chair, or stand while holding the back of a chair. Moving your right foot, make five circles in the air in a clockwise direction, and then make five circles in the opposite direction. Repeat for the left foot.

Knee Bends

Still in a seated position, or holding the chair back, lift your right leg up several inches behind you and bend the leg so that your foot comes toward you slowly. If you are able, lift the foot up behind you. Exhale as you perform this motion, and then inhale as the foot returns to the front and center. Repeat five times. Repeat with the left leg.

The Stepping Warm-Ups

Because T'ai Chi movements include a stepping pattern that is perhaps unique to this art, it would serve us well to practice this particular walking style. The following warm-up gets you up and moving, gets the blood circulating and the synapses in your brain firing, and improves your balance and your kinesthetic sense. (Your kinesthetic sense is your sense of where your body is in relation to the ground and objects around you. If you are the type of person who constantly bumps into things, your kinesthetic sense may need some refining.)

Cat Stepping: Step by Step

Called "Cat Stepping," this is the basic leg technique in T'ai Chi. It is designed to enable you to turn in any direction while maintaining your alignment, and also serves to strengthen both your leg muscles and your sense of balance. In this exercise, you'll learn and practice basic T'ai Chi body mechanics.

Start from a neutral standing position—feet shoulder-width apart and parallel, knees slightly bent, pelvis tipped forward and slightly upward, head lifted, shoulders relaxed. Consider that you are standing on the face of a giant clock and that you are currently standing in the center, facing 12 o'clock.

We will start by stepping out with our right foot toward 2 o'clock (approximately 45 degrees to the right). If done properly, the right leg is now slightly ahead of the left and is pointed out slightly to the right. Now for the left foot. Bring it up directly next to the right foot, and then proceed to step out to the 10 o'clock position. Again, the left foot should now be slightly ahead of the right and pointed outward. The angle between the two feet at this point should be about 90 degrees.

The actual mechanics of the stepping are what is really important, as well as the alignment of the body both during and after the step. You want to feel as though you are ice-skating as you perform this exercise—the legs move in a flowing, circular path. Don't walk stiff-legged like Frankenstein! Let the knees bend, and keep your center of gravity low by imagining a weight attached to your hips, pulling your lower body downward toward the ground. Not too much, or you'll be doing a duck-walk! Be aware of exactly where your balance point is at all times. If you have leg problems, or are not sure of your balance, you can practice this exercise while holding on to a wall. Take small steps—don't try to cover too much ground at one time. Slow and easy does it.

Progress and Safety

You should notice a definite progress forward during your movements. If you are still in your original starting position, then you are doing something not quite right.

Now for an important technique of balance: When you finish a step, pause and look down at your feet. If you were to draw the foot you just stepped with directly back on a straight toe-to-heel line against your other foot, your heels should meet. Often, people will take a "ballet" step, with the feet splayed apart and the heels pointing away from each other. This is fine if you're a ballet dancer, but in T'ai Chi we seek balance, not style. So while you're learning this exercise, pause occasionally and perform this little test to ensure that your alignment is correct.

Also, keeping the knees bent is an important consideration. Just like many buildings in Japan and San Francisco are designed to ride with an earthquake by swaying rather than standing tall and stiff and then crumbling, so too should your knees absorb any minor tremors or shakes that your less-than-perfect balance creates. This also serves to exercise the patellar (kneecap) region.

The weight of your body should drop down through your hips and thighs, passing through the knees, and finally down into the feet. The point at which the weight finally makes contact with the floor, a point approximately midway along the sole of the foot, is called the "Bubbling Spring" point in Chinese medicine.

The proper use and care of the knee joint is also very important. It is well to remember that the knee is a weight-transferal joint, not a weight-bearing one. It is designed to flex only so far without discomfort and damage. So, your weight should pass through the knee without ending there. One way of accomplishing this is to ensure that, during all of your exercises, the kneecap does not move beyond the toes. If you were to hold a yardstick pressed against your big toe perfectly vertical, your knee should not pass that line. This same alignment principle applies to all T'ai Chi and Qigong exercises.

Also in regard to the knee, it is essential that the joint bends directly over the toes, and does not move outward (bowlegged) or inward (knock-kneed), because either condition leads to more knee pain and alignment problems. In the course of your movements, pause occasionally and check that the knees are properly placed, and you'll enjoy many, many years of pain-free T'ai Chi.

Finally, when you are ready to perform the Qigong or T'ai Chi exercises, take a minute and perform an inventory of your starting alignment. The important points are:

- ∽ Feet placed parallel, about shoulder-width apart.
- ∽ Knees slightly bent, but not beyond the toes.
- ∽ Pelvis tilted slightly forward and upward.
- ∽ Head lifted up as if supported by a string.
- ∽ Shoulders, arms, wrists, and fingers relaxed.
- ∽ Tip of tongue placed lightly on roof of mouth, just behind front teeth.

When you are ready to start the exercises, these are the body mechanics you should aim to achieve. Remember to remain soft. There should be no hard lines in the body, every body part is relaxed, yet supported and balanced. This manner of standing may, for some, seem strange and uncomfortable at first, due to years of misalignment and injuries. Keep at it, doing a little bit more each day, and before you know it, you'll feel and look much better.

In the course of performing the Qigong exercises in Chapter 6, there will be times when you are required to pivot one foot outward in order to complete the exercise. When you do this pivot, always attempt to pivot on the heel, not the toe.

This ensures proper alignment and reduces the chance of strain. Also be sure to take the weight off of the foot before pivoting—this is another one of those important principles to watch out for. It ensures that you are not grinding the foot into the floor, that the joints are relaxed and flowing as you execute the pivot, and that you are totally relaxed throughout the movement.

Chapter 6

Flow Like a River

Qigong Exercises

18-Movement Qigong Form

How This Form Will Help You

The 18-Movement Qigong Form contains a good selection of light, gentle movements characteristic of Qigong, done in a slow, graceful manner so that breathing, body position, and mental activity are naturally coordinated. In spite of its simple structure and easy movements, the exercise has proven effective in curing various kinds of chronic ailments, and is particularly suitable for seniors and those with weak constitutions.

It is not only widely practiced in China, but is also increasing in popularity in some Southeast Asian countries, as well as in Japan, Europe, Australia, and the United States.

For those regularly engaged in T'ai Chi practice, the 18-Movement Qigong Form may help them achieve better results from their practice through better co-ordination of breathing, body posture, and mental activity.

This form, created in the 1950s in China, is a wonderful series of movements designed to work your joints, muscles, internal organs, and energy system. It is a useful form for relaxation and stretching, can be adapted to seated or even prone positions (see Chapter 8), and can be used as a learning vehicle for subsequent Qigong forms. This has always been the first Qigong form taught to students in my schools.

Specific areas worked in this form include wrists, shoulders, neck, torso/spine, waist, knees, and ankles. The benefits of each movement in the form is explained in the instructions for that movement.

Each of these forms can be performed from one to 100 times, depending on your agility, breathing rate, and available time. However many repetitions you perform, and however many of the forms you do, you should practice at least once per day, for 15 minutes minimum. The more you practice, the greater the benefits will be.

Remember to breathe diaphragmatically, through the nose on both inhale and exhale. This is the key to generating Qi.

Tips for Performing

As in all Qigong and T'ai Chi forms, it pays to remember several important points in order to make your practice both easier and more effective.

First, remember your posture and alignment. Posture will be straight but not stiff, with the head lifted at the crown as if a string were pulling it upward. Be sure not to tilt or sway the head during the exercises. The pelvis will be tilted slightly forward and upward—not as if you're doing an Elvis impression—only very slightly. The feet are approximately shoulder-width and parallel. The knees are slightly bent.

The shoulders should be relaxed at the beginning of the form. In the course of performing the movements, some may require a lifting of the shoulders. This should be accomplished with as little strain and effort as possible. The elbows are always slightly bent, never locked. The fingers are curled naturally, slightly inward toward the palm.

The gaze is level and relaxed, the tip of the tongue is resting lightly on the roof of the mouth, just behind the upper incisors. The chin is tucked slightly in—not enough to alter the alignment of the head, but just enough so that you don't tilt the head backward.

The breathing is, hopefully, diaphragmatic and slow. When you first start to practice these movements, your mind will be occupied with getting the movements right, so just breathe naturally. You can add in the proper breathing techniques later.

Note: Form names preceded by an asterisk (*) are names that I have given to the movements to allow easier recall and visualization. The traditional visualization for each form is listed first, followed by my alternate representation, also preceded by an asterisk (*).

Form 1
Starting Position—Opening—Origin
(*Riding the Tide)

Stand at ease with feet parallel and shoulder-width apart, trunk upright, eyes looking straight ahead, chest relaxed and slightly concave, back lifted, hands hanging at the sides [Photos 1 and 2].

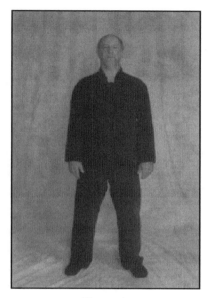

Photo 1.

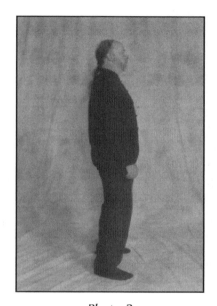

Photo 2.

1. Inhale as you slowly lift arms forward to shoulder level with palms facing downward [Photo 3].

2. Keeping trunk upright, exhale as you bend knees until thighs form an angle of about 150 degrees with lower legs and press palms down to abdomen level. Knees should not go beyond the tips of the toes.

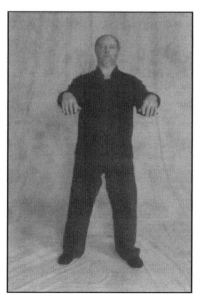

Photo 3.

Points for Attention:

Sink shoulders and drop elbows when you move your arms, with fingers naturally flexed, and with body weight resting on both feet. Do *not* allow your buttocks to protrude when you bend knees. The pressing down of palms should be coordinated with the bending of knees. Inhale and exhale with nose. This breathing method should be applied in all the forms of this exercise.

Visualization:

Imagine yourself rising and falling smoothly like the water shooting from a fountain.

*Imagine you are floating upright in the ocean, with your hands and arms gently rising and falling with the waves.

Effects:

The rise and fall of the body helps activate the flow of Qi, unblock the energy passages and regulate Qi and blood. It is good for ailments such as high blood pressure, heart disease, and hepatitis. Those suffering from these ailments can do this form as a separate exercise, in which the movements may be performed as many times as suits the condition of the individual. The same can be said of all other forms in this exercise.

Form 2
Opening the Chest (*Gimme a Hug!)

1. Lift both arms forward to chest level, while inhaling, with palms facing downward, then turn your palms so that the thumbs point upward before moving arms horizontally to the sides to expand chest and continuing the inhale [Photo 4].

2. Exhale and bring hands toward each other and turn palms downward when they are held in front of your chest. Continue to exhale as you press palms downward to original position.

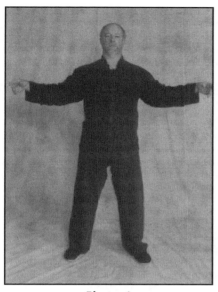

Photo 4.

Points for Attention:

Straighten up gradually as you lift arms in front of chest, and bend knees slightly as you press palms downward. These movements should be performed with continuity and co-ordinated with breathing.

Visualization:

Imagine yourself standing on the top of a high mountain and looking far into the distance with a tranquil mind.

*Imagine you meet a friend you haven't seen in years, and you open your arms wide to hug them.

Effects:

Good for pulmonary emphysema, heart disease, shortness of breath, palpitation, chest distress, neurasthenia, and neurosis.

Form 3
Painting the Rainbow

1. Start inhaling as you slowly straighten knees and lift arms up to chest level with palms facing down.

2. Keep inhaling as you do the following movements: Move arms up overhead while shifting weight onto right foot with right knee slightly bent, left leg straightened and turned 90 degrees outward to the left; then, lower left arm parallel to the floor on the left side with palm up [Photo 5].

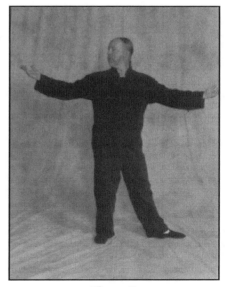

Photo 5.

3. While exhaling, the bent right arm will now "paint a rainbow," or move in a circular fashion overhead and to the stationary left palm. When the palms are 3 inches apart, both hands form a "ball" or circular-holding shape [Photo 6] and continue down to in front of the abdomen. The weight has remained on the bent right leg until the hands reach the abdomen, then the left foot turns back to the front position, the weight is centered on both legs, and the hands begin the same movement again as Step 1, this time to the opposite side [Photos 7 and 8].

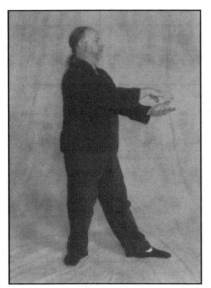

Photo 6.

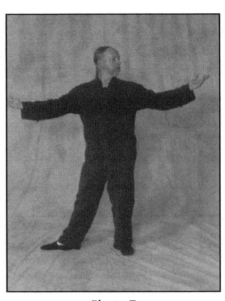

Photo 7.

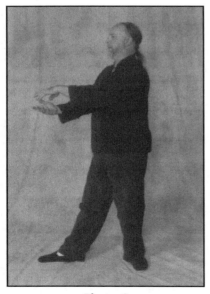

Photo 8.

Points for Attention:

The "painting" of the arms should be gracefully coordinated with breathing and with the lifting of the arms.

Visualization:

Imagine yourself painting a rainbow above your head.

Effects:

This form helps take off fat from the midsection and is good for backache and kidney diseases.

Form 4
Parting the Clouds

1. Center the weight on both legs. Lower both arms and cross hands in front of lower abdomen, palms facing inward [Photo 9].

2. Inhale as the arms pivot upward, keeping the palms facing your body, until the hands are overhead [Photo 10].

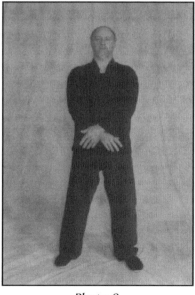

Photo 9.

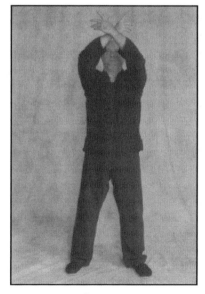

Photo 10.

3. Exhale and turn the wrists so that the palms now face outward (backs of hands are facing each other) [Photo 11] and move the arms outward and downward in a gentle arc [Photo 12]. Continue the downward motion until the hands are once again crossed in front of the lower abdomen.

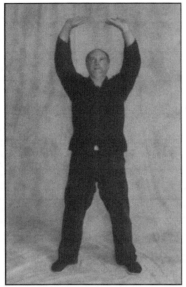

Photo 11.

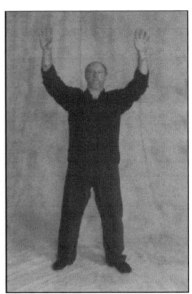

Photo 12.

Points for Attention:

Use shoulder joints as rotational points when you swing arms up, lifting chin slightly and expanding the chest as you inhale. Relax the shoulders as the hands descend.

Visualization:

Imagine yourself thrusting your hands into the clouds, then grabbing the edges of the hole that you made and pulling the clouds apart.

Effects:

This form helps generate Qi and build up strength in the waist and legs, and is good for heart disease, shortness of breath, and periarthritis of the shoulder.

Form 5
Whirling Arms on Horseback
(*Plate of Spaghetti)

1. With feet remaining in normal stance (shoulder-width), inhale; lift both hands up to shoulder level in front of the body, palms facing downward.

2. Still inhaling, shift the weight to the right leg, bending the right knee, and bring the right hand up to the right shoulder, fingers facing backward and palm facing up.

3. Still inhaling, extend the left arm to the left, with a slight bend in the elbow, fingers pointing to the left and palm up.

4. Finally, still inhaling, turn the head and gaze to the left, past the extended left hand [Photo 13].

5. Now exhale and bring the body weight to a 50/50 distribution, while bringing both hands together in front of the chest and "squeezing a meatball," or holding an imaginary ball with the hands. At the same time, the head and torso return to the front [Photo 14].

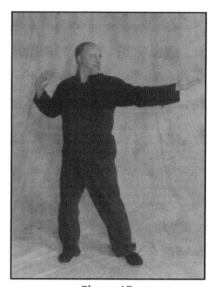

Photo 13.

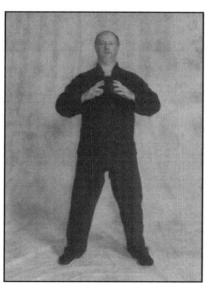

Photo 14.

6. Repeat these movements to the opposite side [Photo 15].

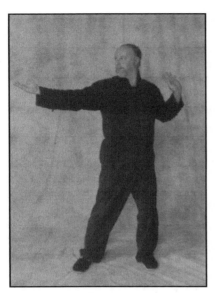

Photo 15.

Points for Attention:

Palms should be as flat as possible when "holding the plate of spaghetti." Fix your gaze into the distance as you look past your outstretched hand.

Visualization:

You vigorously whirl your arms while riding a horse.

*You are a waiter(ess) in a busy restaurant, balancing a plate of spaghetti on your shoulder and pointing across the room to the tables. The cook put too much sauce on the pasta, it's too heavy, so your leg begins to bend a little on that side. You dropped the plate! Then you start making meatballs to go with the next order of spaghetti.

Effects:

Good for inflammation in the shoulder, elbow, and wrist joints and for asthma, trachitis, and kidney diseases.

Form 6
Rowing on the Lake

1. From the end of the previous movement (holding an imaginary ball at chest level), let both arms drop to the sides of the body and bend knees slightly [Photo 16].

2. Bringing the arms backward and upward, begin raising the arms until they are overhead, palms facing forward [Photo 17]. Allow the arms to drop slowly down, palms down, while bending the knees.

3. This movement is repeated continuously, effecting a rowing, or "butterfly stroke," motion. Inhale on the upswing and exhale on the downward movement.

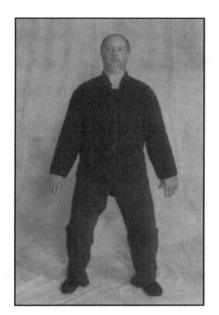

Photo 16.

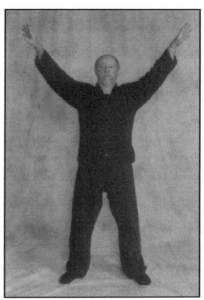

Photo 17.

Points for Attention:

Keep the back straight when descending and keep the gaze level.

Visualization:

You are slowly swimming on a calm lake.

Effects:

This form helps improve the function of the digestive system and is good for gastrointestinal ailments, heart disease, and neurasthenia.

Form 7
Holding a Ball at Shoulder Level
(*Scooping the Ice Cream)

1. At the completion of Form 6, return to a starting position. Scoop with the right hand across the body to the left and upward, as if scooping up a ball, and hold the palm up at shoulder level [Photo 18].

2. Drop the right hand back down to your right side, and repeat the movement with the left hand toward the right side of the body. Inhale as the hand drops down, exhale as the hand scoops [Photo 19].

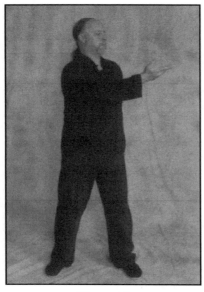

Photo 18.

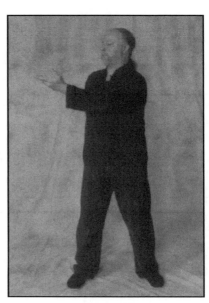

Photo 19.

Points for Attention:

Look at the "ball" you are imagining to be holding, and keep the shoulders relaxed.

Visualization:

Imagine you are a young child, gleefully playing with a ball.

*You were fired from that restaurant because of the spaghetti incident, so now you're scooping ice cream, vanilla with the right hand and chocolate with the left.

Effects:

Increases coordination and balance, works the shoulder joints and wrist joints.

Form 8
Gazing at the Moon Over the Shoulder

1. At the completion of Form 7, return to a starting position.

2. Swing the arms backward, upward, and to the left while turning the trunk in coordination, turning the head as if to look at the moon, and exhale. The left arm is outstretched and pointing at the moon, the right hand is palm up beneath the left armpit [Photo 20].

3. Swing both arms down and repeat to the right side of the body [Photo 21]. Inhale as the arms swing down; exhale as you gaze at the moon.

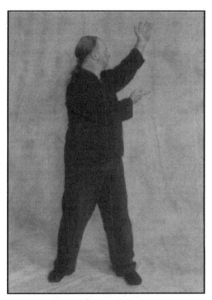

Photo 20.

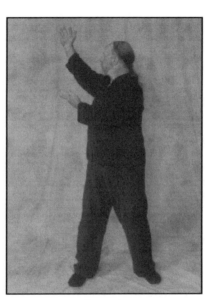

Photo 21.

Points for Attention:

The arms, trunk, and head should all move as a single unit.

Visualization:

Imagine you are pointing out the magnificent moon to a friend.

*Just a little aside here: I usually see Ralph Cramden's face on the moon.

Effects:

Good for the lower and upper back, shoulders, and neck. This form has helped many of my students who are golfers. Just remember, in *this* exercise, keep your head UP.

Form 9
Press Palms Across the Body

1. After completing Form 8, return to a starting position. Press the right palm, fingers pointing up, across your stomach and to the left side of the body, keeping the

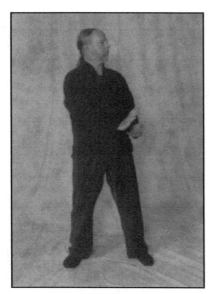

right arm close to the body. Meanwhile, the left hand "parks" on the left side, palm up with the little finger touching the side of the body and the fingers pointing forward [Photo 22]. Bring the hands back to a central position with the palms facing upward and fingers pointing at each other [Photo 23].

Photo 22.

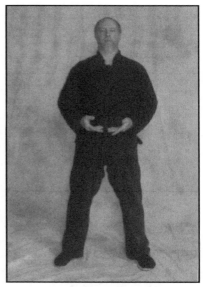

Photo 23.

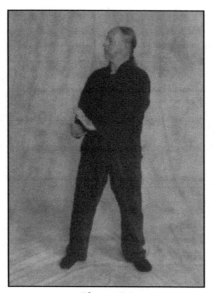

2. Repeat this movement in the opposite direction, with the left hand pressing and the right hand parking [Photo 24].

Photo 24.

Points for Attention:

Keep the arms close to the body and low on the torso. Relax the shoulders. Exhale as you press; inhale as the hands pass your middle. Turn only the waist, NOT the hips, as you press across your body.

Visualization:

Imagine you are slowly pressing against two walls that are pressing in on you. Move the hands as if there is a short length of string tied to both wrists, so that they move in unison.

Effects:

This form is good for toning the waist muscles and learning to use minimal effort.

Form 10
Wave Hands Like Clouds
(*The Non-Attachment Exercise)

1. From a neutral stance, begin circling the left hand counterclockwise, keeping the palm facing the body [Photo 25]. As the left hand passes in front of the face, the right hand is slowly being pulled across the lower abdomen to the left by virtue

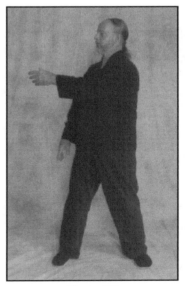

Photo 25.

of the body turning to the left [Photos 26 and 27]. As both arms arrive at the left side of your body, drop the left arm down and raise the right arm [Photo 28].

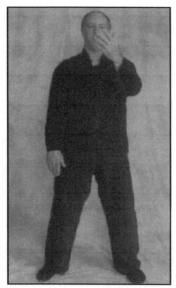

Photo 26.

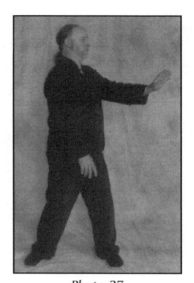

Photo 27.

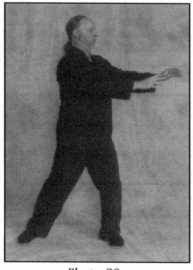

Photo 28.

2. Now circle the right hand clockwise, again keeping the palm toward the body at face level, as the left arm is allowed to pass across the lower abdomen [Photos 29 through 32]. Continue circling both arms in opposite directions.

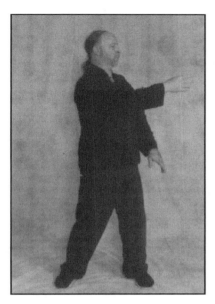

Photo 29.

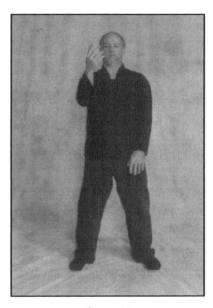

Photo 30.

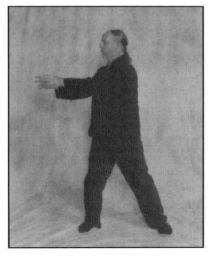

Photo 31.

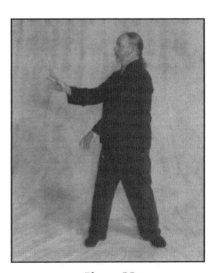

Photo 32.

Points for Attention:

Use the body to pull the hands across, don't just wave your arms, but propel them with the body turning. Keep the bottom hand relaxed. Inhale as the left hand passes the face; exhale as the right hand passes the face.

Visualization:

Your hands are drifting by like clouds.

*Each Qigong movement has a little clue contained within it, which an expert can decipher and use to gauge the psychological makeup of the student performing the movement. Wave Hands Like Clouds falls into the "non-attachment" category—if the bottom hand in the movement is stiff and bent, that usually indicates that the student is "holding on" to a grievance or other powerful emotion.

Effects:

This form is good for neurasthenia, gastrointestinal disorders, and indigestion. It also helps enliven the brain and improve memory.

Form 11
Scoop the Sea and Look to the Sky
(*Pick Up the Shells and Throw 'Em in the Air)

1. Step out and forward 45 degrees with your left leg. Putting approximately 70 percent of your body weight on the left leg, bend forward and downward over the leg and scoop up with both hands [Photo 33].

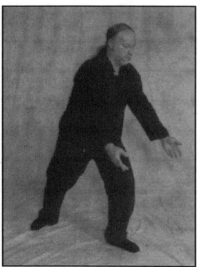

Photo 33.

2. Shift your weight back to your right leg, lift up your left toes, raise your head to look up, and open up your arms, palms upward, as you lean back as far as comfortable [Photo 34].

Points for Attention:

Keep the right foot flat at all times. Inhale as you scoop, and exhale as you lean back.

Visualization:

You are slowly scooping up water from the seashore, and then looking up in the air.

*Just for fun, you're scooping up seashells and throwing them in the air.

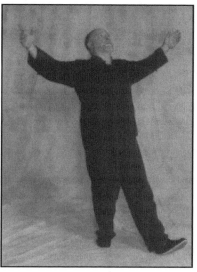

Photo 34.

Effects:

Helps strengthen the kidneys and spleen and develops strength in the legs and waist.

Form 12
Set the Waves Rolling (*Push the Refrigerator)

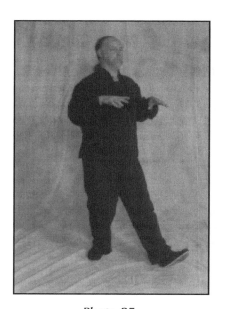

Photo 35.

1. After the last "looking up" movement from Form 11, level your head, drop your hands to chest height, and lower your elbows [Photo 35].

2. Shift forward 70 percent onto your left leg while pushing forward and upward at chest-level with both hands. The fingers should point up during the push [Photo 36].

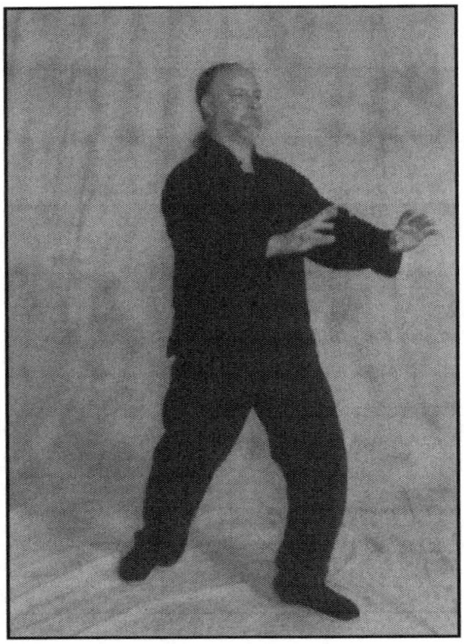

3. Roll back, or shift your weight back onto your right leg while lifting your left toes, and withdraw both hands to your chest.

4. The hands, while shifting forward to push, create a semicircular path: starting from the chest, dropping toward the abdomen as they go forward, and ending once again at chest level, as if you are tracing the bottom of a bowl with your fingertips.

Points for Attention:

Keep the right foot flat at all times. Inhale as you roll back and exhale as you push.

Photo 36.

Visualization:

You are gently rolling back and forth, like waves at the beach.

*You are moving the refrigerator to clean the floor underneath it. What, you mean you don't do that?!

Effects:

Good for hepatitis, pulmonary disease, neuralgia, neurasthenia, and insomnia.

Form 13
Dove Spreads Wings

1. After the last push from Form 12, the hands are palm forward at chest level, and the weight is 70 percent on the left leg.

2. Turn the palms to face each other, fingers pointing forward. Shift your weight back onto your right leg and open your arms outward, to the sides of your body, keeping the thumbs up [Photo 37].

3. Shift the weight forward again, and close the arms forward until the palms are almost touching [Photo 38].

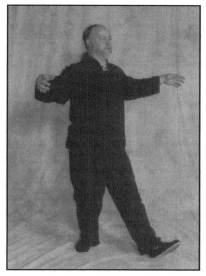

Photo 37.

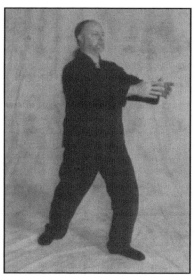

Photo 38.

Points for Attention:

Inhale as you open your arms and exhale as you close. Keep the right foot flat at all times.

Visualization:

Imagine you are a dove spreading its wings and breathing in fresh air.

Effects:

Effective for curing chest distress, and pulmonary and heart diseases.

Form 14
Punching From a Horseback Riding Stance
(*Punch With Two Fists)

1. Assume a horseback riding stance with the hands formed into fists, palms up, at the sides of the body [Photo 39].

2. Punch forward with the right fist, turning the fist over as you do so (corkscrew punch), at chest level [Photo 40].

3. Bring the right fist back to the side, and repeat with the left fist [Photo 41].

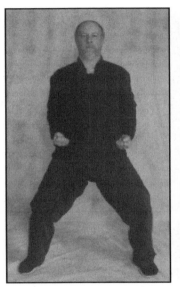 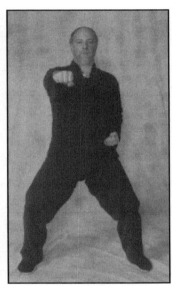 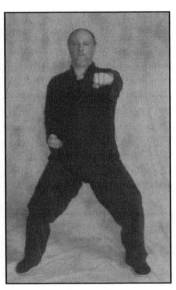

Photo 39. Photo 40. Photo 41.

Points for Attention:

Exhale as you punch and inhale as you return. Keep the knees bent and the back straight.

Visualization:

You should feel like a martial artist toughening your body.

*This is a great stress reliever. Imagine that you are facing someone or something that has caused you trouble, and really tear into them. But remember: go slowly!

Effects:

Adds to your internal strength, and helps cultivate primordial Qi. It is good for asthma, bronchitis, and neurosis.

Form 15
Wild Goose in Flight

1. Return to a shoulder-width stance, knees slightly bent, and drop arms to sides.

2. Raise arms sideways to slightly above shoulder level, palms down, and lift your heels up [Photo 42].

3. Drop your arms down to your sides and lower your heels.

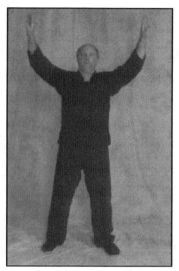

Points for Attention:

Keep the wrist joints flexible. The rise and fall of the heels, arms, and body should all be coordinated with the breathing—inhale as you go up and exhale as you come down. If you can't lift the heels without losing your balance, just flap your wings.

Visualization:

Imagine sailing freely in the sky like a large goose. (Honking is optional, but strongly recommended.)

Photo 42.

Effects:

Helps remove mental strain and is good for vertigo, fullness of the head, and nervous disorders.

Form 16
Turning the Windmill

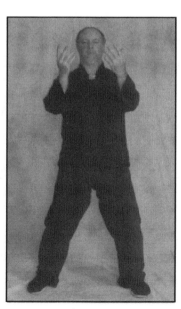

1. Keeping the arms slightly bent at the elbows, turn them in giant circles, first counterclockwise, then clockwise [Photo 43].

2. The palms face the body at both face level and lower abdomen level.

Photo 43.

Points for Attention:

Inhale as your arms circle beneath waist level; exhale as they pass across at face level. Shift your weight side to side and turn your waist and hips to propel the arms.

Visualization:

Imagine that you are a giant windmill turning slowly in a breeze.

Effects:

Stimulates the flow of blood and Qi, enlivens one's spirits, and is good for arthritis and obesity.

Form 17
Marching in Place While Bouncing the Ball

1. Lift left knee and raise right arm to waist height, then lower right hand as if bouncing a ball while setting left foot down [Photo 44].

2. Repeat with right knee and left arm and hand [Photo 45].

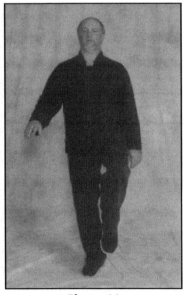

Photo 44.

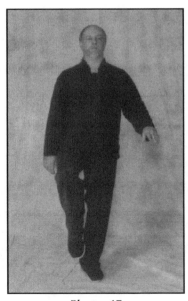

Photo 45.

Points for Attention:

Inhale as you raise your knee; exhale as you set it down. Align your body over your supporting leg, which is kept slightly bent. Fix your gaze forward and level. Be sure not to do the Rockettes variation, where you lift your leg and pull it across your opposite leg. Make sure you lift it straight up, as if lifting with a string.

Visualization:

You are a young child gleefully playing with a ball while marching in place.

Effects:

Helps remove fatigue and restore physical strength; improves balance.

Form 18
Press Palms and Calm Down (*Closing)

1. Hold a ball at the level of the lower abdomen, and lift it up to chest level [Photos 46 and 47].

2. Turn both palms downward and gently press down until the hands are at your sides [Photo 48].

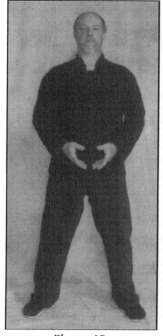
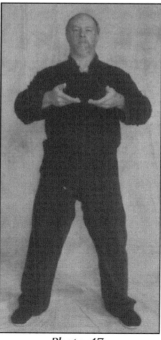
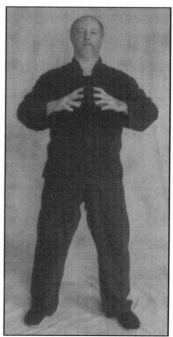

Photo 46.   *Photo 47.*   *Photo 48.*

Points for Attention:

Keep the gaze relaxed. Keep the shoulders down. Inhale as you lift; exhale as you press down.

Effects:

This form produces a tranquilizing effect and is good for high blood pressure and heart disease. Every good Qigong form has a finishing movement that is designed to calm you down after your workout and put your energy away, much like a child putting away her toys when she's done playing.

Adaptations

Adapting the 18-Movement Qigong Form is quite easily done, and is useful for both the wheelchair-bound student and the student with leg problems such as poor circulation or arthritic joints.

If you are seated, make sure that your head is still suspended by that imaginary string. A properly aligned spine and neck are vital to achieving the benefits that are offered by these exercises. If possible, sit with both feet flat on the floor. Because balance will generally not be an issue when performing seated exercises, you are able to concentrate more on the hand movements and their associated breathing patterns.

Of course, the hand movements themselves will be slightly modified to allow easy movement. As a general rule, if in performing the standing version of the movement, the hands and arms descend below the waist, in the seated version they will glide across the lap. So in a movement such as Wave Hands Like Clouds, for instance, the bottom hand will simply move horizontally over the thighs, while the top hand still glides across at face level.

The feet do not turn or pivot as they do in the standing version, nor do you shift weight from leg to leg. The waist, however, is still used to initiate all movements. This style of performance places more emphasis on spinal flexibility and lower-back muscle development.

For the three movements performed in the standing version with one leg extended (Pick Up the Shells, Push the Refrigerator, and Dove Spreads Wings), simply spread the legs slightly apart when performing the seated version.

For more detailed information on how to perform these movements from a seated position, see Chapter 8.

The Eight Pieces of Brocade

How This Form Will Help You

The Eight Pieces of Brocade is a much older Qigong exercise, hailing from 12th-century China. Said to have been invented by Marshall Yeuh Fei to improve the health of his soldiers, this form serves to strengthen both muscles and bones through its often-martial poses. Within the eight movements of this form are three that employ the horseback riding stance. Remember to go only as wide in this stance as your balance and leg strength allow.

The eight movements will strengthen the kidneys, stomach, liver, spleen, lungs, and heart. In addition, it develops your *shen*, or spirit, through the act of vigorously punching an imaginary opponent; works upon eliminating emotional distress such as anger, sorrow, and hate; and serves to eliminate temporary afflictions such as heartburn and indigestion.

Tips for Performing

The same precautions and hints outlined in the 18-Movement Qigong Form apply here as well: straight yet relaxed posture, feet shoulder-width and parallel, knees slightly bent, head suspended, pelvis tucked, and shoulders relaxed.

This set of principles applies to any and all T'ai Chi and Qigong exercises that you will ever do, so it's a good time to indelibly mark them in your brain.

The Eight Pieces of Brocade Qigong Form

Note: For each movement, in addition to the traditional name and the name I regularly use for my students, I am including another Chinese variation, the title of which is preceded by two asterisks (**), to illustrate first, how confusing the terminology can become, and second, to make you laugh! These are actual translations from a Chinese Qigong class I attended many years ago.

First Movement
Double Hands Hold Up the Heavens
(*Two Hands Hold Up the Sky)
(**Lift Two Arms Up to Sky-Height, Be Your Gut in Great Delight)

Stand in a neutral position with your feet parallel and shoulder-width apart, with your hands at your sides. Close your eyes, calm your mind, and breathe deeply and regularly. Open your eyes, gaze straight forward, continue breathing naturally and smoothly. Inhale, interlock your fingers, palms up in front of your lower abdomen [Photo 49], and raise your hands above your head while slightly bending your elbows [Photo 50].

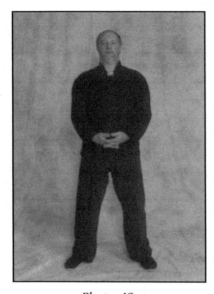

Photo 49.

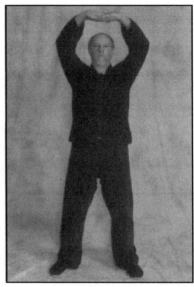

Photo 50.

Exhale, tip or tilt your body to the left [Photo 51], and then stand straight up again while inhaling. Tilt to the right [Photo 52], then stand up straight again. Do not lower your hands down in front of your body until you are finished with as many repetitions as you wish to perform.

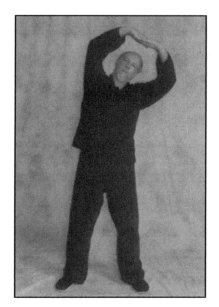

Photo 51.

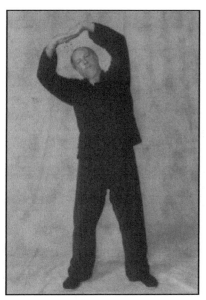

Photo 52.

Effects: This movement works with an area called the *Sanjiao,* or Triple Burner. The three areas of the Triple Burner are: above the diaphragm, between the diaphragm and navel, and between the navel and the groin. These three burners are said to control, respectively, respiration, digestion, and elimination, and also act as the body's thermostat. So if you're prone to hot flashes, or constantly feel cold, this is the form for you.

Second Movement
Aim the Bow and Shoot the Arrow
(**Shooting the Hawk by Drawing the Bow Tight,
Do This Twice With Your Left and Right)

Step out into a horseback riding stance. Bring your hands together at your lower abdomen level as if holding a small ball. Raise the ball to chest level [Photo 53]. Shift your weight to your right leg and turn your torso to face the right side. Extend the hands to the right side, the right hand extending out, index and middle finger pointing at your "target"; the left hand, formed into a fist, pulling the imaginary string [Photo 54].

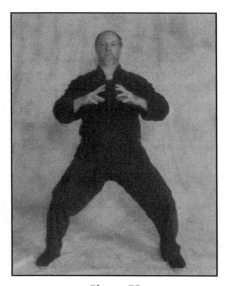

Photo 53.

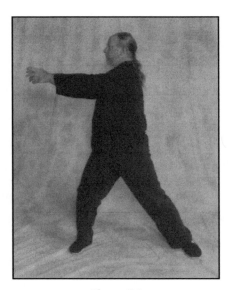

Photo 54.

Pull the bowstring taut, back to the center of your chest, tensing both hands and arms [Photo 55], then release the "arrow" and relax the arms and hands. Bring both hands back in front of the body at chest level, forming a ball. Repeat on the left side [Photos 56 and 57] to complete one repetition.

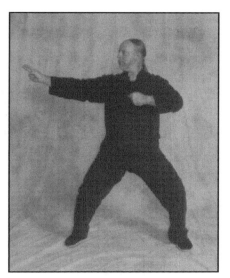

Photo 55.

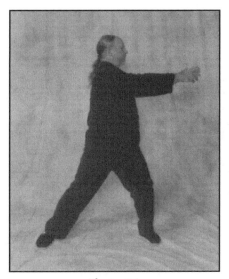

Photo 56.

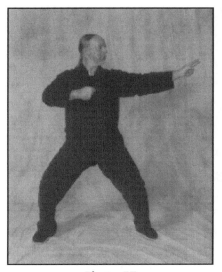

Photo 57.

Effects: This movement is used to strengthen the kidneys and the waist area. First you must sink down, to root yourself as when you pull a strong bow. Without this root, you will not have strong balance, and will not be able to pull the bow effectively. Make sure that when you squat down, you keep your back straight and tuck your buttocks under. This places emphasis on the kidneys. When you do this, you not only strengthen the waist muscles, but also increase the Qi circulation in the kidney area. Focus your mind so that you really feel that you are drawing a very strong bow. This focused mind is one of the key benefits of this movement: developing your ability to concentrate.

Third Movement
Alternately Supporting Heaven and Earth
(**If You Wish Your Spleen and Stomach All Right, Be One Arm of Yours Raised up and Stretched Tight)

After the last movement, return to a neutral stance and move both hands to the front of your body at stomach level, with your palms facing up [Photo 58]. Lift your left hand above your head, palm facing up, and push up. At the same time, lower your right hand, palm down, and push downward [Photo 59]. Then change hands and repeat the same movements [Photo 60]. You should imagine that the hands are pushing against both the sky and the earth, but do not push with the muscles. Push instead with your Qi.

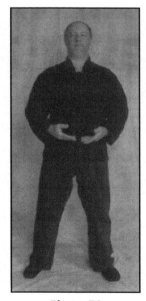
Photo 58.

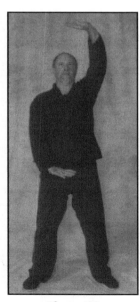
Photo 59.

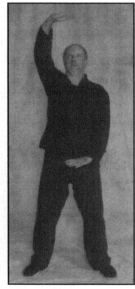
Photo 60.

Effects: This movement works the stomach. When you repeatedly raise one hand and lower the other, you loosen the muscles in the front of the body. When you push with the palms, do not tense the muscles, but rather extend your force through the hands so that your arms stretch out, remembering to keep the elbows slightly bent. This stimulates and strengthens the tendons and muscles. Reversing your arms repeatedly stretches and relaxes the body, "waking up" the tendons. This type of muscle movement increases the Qi circulation in the stomach, spleen, and liver.

Fourth Movement
Five Weaknesses and Seven Injuries Disappear
(*Look Behind You!)
(**Look Backwards as Much as You Might,
Will Recover Your Body From Tiredness Quite)

Stand in a neutral position as before, hands hanging naturally at your sides. Turn your head to the left and exhale [Photo 61], then return your head to the front as you inhale. Turn your head to the right and exhale [Photo 62], then return to the front and inhale. Repeat as many times as desired. Your body should remain facing the front.

Next, place your hands on your waist, thumbs facing forward and palms upward, and turn your head as before [Photo 63]. Do not turn your body when you look to the rear.

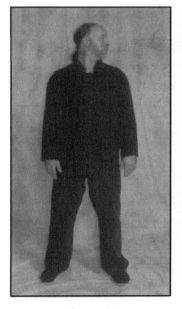
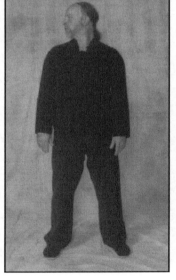
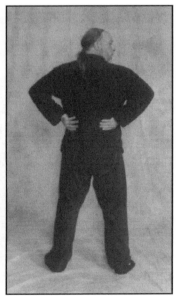

Photo 61.   Photo 62.   Photo 63.

Finally, move both hands to your chest, palms facing up, press your elbows and shoulders slightly forward, and turn your head as before [Photo 64].

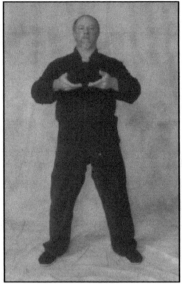

Photo 64.

Effects: Five Weaknesses in Traditional Chinese Medicine refers to illnesses of the five yin organs: heart, liver, spleen, lungs, and kidneys. The Seven Injuries refers to injuries caused by emotions: happiness, anger, sorrow, joy, love, hate, and desire. According to TCM, you can become ill when your internal organs are weak, and emotional disturbance upsets them. For example, excessive sorrow can cause the Qi in your heart to stagnate, which will affect the functioning of the organ. But your organs are not the only things affected: Strong emotions also cause Qi to accumulate in your head. When you turn your head from side to side, you loosen up the muscles, blood vessels, and Qi channels in your neck, and allow the Qi in your head to smooth out. In addition, there is a physical release of tension and stress that is carried there.

Fifth Movement
Sway the Head and Swing the Tail
(**By Turning Your Head and Wagging Your Butt
To a Degree Finite, Your Ill-Temper Will Say, "Good Night")

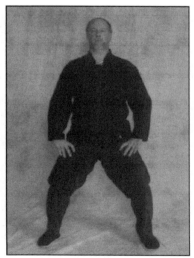

Photo 65.

Move your right leg out about 1 foot to the right, and sink into a horseback riding stance. Place your hands on top of your knees, with the thumbs facing backwards [Photo 65]. Shift your weight to your left leg, and press down with your left hand, while attempting to bend your head and spine over the left leg [Photo 66]. Stay in this position for three seconds, and then return to the center. Repeat on the opposite side [Photo 67]. Inhale through the center; exhale when pressing to the sides. Make sure when you lean that you don't tilt your head; keep a straight line.

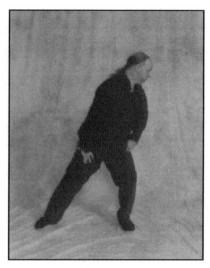

Photo 66.

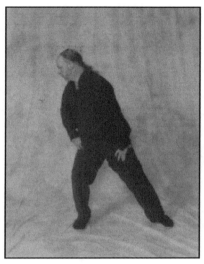

Photo 67.

Effects: This exercise "extinguishes fire in the heart." Translated, this means that if you have heartburn, or suffer from breathing impure air or from lack of sleep, this exercise will help you. It works the lungs like bellows, and allows the Qi to pass from the Middle Tan Tien—or the heart and lung region—through any obstructions.

Sixth Movement
Lift and Touch Toes
(*Push the Sky and Reach
Down to the Ground)
(**Touch the Tip-Toes With Your Left
and Right, Be Your Waist In Good Sight)

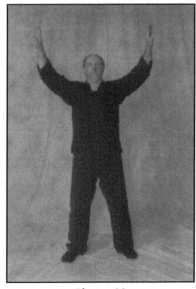

Move your right leg back to its original position (shoulder-width apart). Allow your hands to press palm-down at your sides, and then slowly raise them in front of the chest, palms facing up. Continue to rise until they are "pushing" overhead [Photo 68]. Make sure the elbows are slightly bent at this point, and the shoulders relaxed. Inhale while raising the hands, exhale while pushing upward.

Photo 68.

Now, inhale and drop the hands and arms down, bending at the waist, and reach down as far as is comfortable [Photo 69]. In this movement, the knees are *locked.* Exhale while reaching down for a count of three, and then slowly rise upward, inhaling as you do.

Effects: When you bend forward and reach down, you are stretching the muscles in your back and also restricting the flow of Qi to your kidneys. When you rise up, you release the Qi and remove any blockages from the kidney meridians.

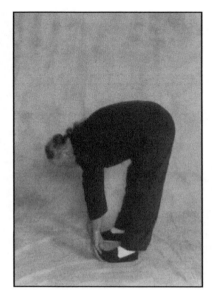

Photo 69.

Seventh Movement
Screw the Fists With Fiery Eyes
(**With Your Fiery Eyesight, as If You're Doing a Fist-Fight; The Way to Develop Your Strength by Making You Excite)

Step with your right foot to the side into a horseback riding stance, forming fists with both hands. The fists are held at belt-level on the sides of the body, palms upward [Photo 70]. Turn your head and glare fiercely to the right, and slowly extend the right arm and fist, turning the fist over as it extends (Also known as a "karate punch") [Photo 71]. Exhale while punching. Now return the fist [Photo 72], inhale, and turn your attention to the left side, extending the left fist and arm in a similar manner [Photo 73]. The opposing fist remains tight and "parked" at your side.

Effects: This movement trains you to raise your spirit, or *Shen.* When your spirit is raised, you strengthen the Qi flow and also increase muscular strength (*Li*). As you increase your Qi-enhanced muscular strength (*Qi Li*), you fill your body with spirit and energy. In the other exercises, you have been focusing your intent and Qi on various parts of the body. It is important to do this piece because it clears out any stagnant Qi and leads it to the skin. Concentrating your mind (*Yi*) is the key to success in this movement; have a strong mental image of punching someone very hard.

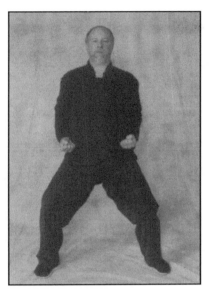

Photo 70.

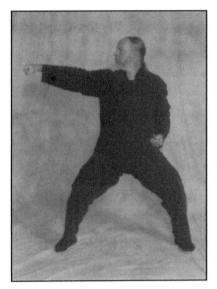

Photo 71.

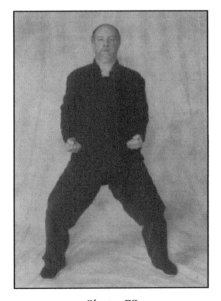

Photo 72.

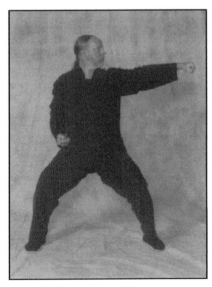

Photo 73.

Eighth Movement
Feet and Head Lifted
(*Lift Your Heels)
(**Seven Times After You Bob Your Heels and Let Them Alight,
No More Illness You Have to Fight)

With the hands comfortably at your sides, push up your entire body by lifting the heels and putting the body's weight on the balls and toes of the feet [Photo 74]. Inhale as your rise up; exhale as you slowly come back down. Keep your knees slightly bent throughout the entire exercise.

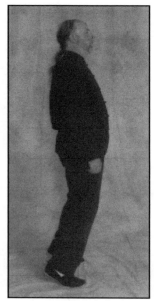

Effects: This movement is used to smooth out the Qi from head to toes. When you lift your heels, you are stimulating six of the main Qi channels in the body, allowing a free flow of energy. When finished with this piece, stand quietly and breathe for a minute or so, remaining calm and aware of your body.

Photo 74.

Adaptations

As with the 18-Movement Qigong Form, adaptations for the Eight Pieces of Brocade are quite simple. There is actually a separate Seated Eight Pieces of Brocade Qigong Form, but it is a bit more advanced than we have the space for in this book.

When performing the Eight Pieces of Brocade sitting down, be aware of the body alignment and posture. Again, recall the basics: feet flat (if, as with some of my students, your feet don't reach the ground when seated, just grab a phone book and place your feet on top of it), head suspended by that invisible string, back straight but not tense.

The first movement that may cause problems is Form 5, Sway the Head and Swing the Tail, as it is difficult to lean over to the side of a chair without losing your balance. Just go slowly, and don't exceed your comfort level. Over time, you'll gain more flexibility and be able to bend further.

The horseback riding stance for Form 7, Screw the Fists With Fiery Eyes, can be accomplished while seated by simply spreading the legs apart as far as is comfortable, remembering to keep the feet parallel and flat.

Form 8, Lift Your Heels, becomes problematic when seated. Simply lift your heels up, hold, and then relax back down. Focus more on the breathing and relaxation aspects of this movement.

Again, more information on seated adaptations will be forthcoming in Chapter 8.

Congratulations! You're now an experienced Qigong player. Now, it's time to investigate T'ai Chi, the "moving meditation" that works on balance and coordination. In the next chapter, we'll introduce you to basic principles of T'ai Chi movement, alignment, and breathing, and we'll practice some exercises to get you firing away on all eight cylinders. Once again, good job!

Chapter 7

Shall We Dance?

Standing T'ai Chi Exercises

A Review of Core T'ai Chi Principles

A review of the basic principles of T'ai Chi movement is in order at this point, because without a firm grasp of these basics, you are not doing T'ai Chi, just a slow-motion dance. With the principles in mind, however, you will enter into the magical world of healing and relaxation, of spiritual cleansing, and of greater everyday optimism.

Starting with your feet, place them shoulder-width apart and parallel. Remember that the feet should be parallel in order to reduce the stress on the ankles and knees, and although you may normally walk splayfooted, at least for the duration of these exercises try to indulge my taste in foot alignment.

The knees should be slightly bent, not as if you are being crushed under a two-ton weight, but comfortably. The main idea is to get away from locking the knees, a common practice in many people. Recall that energy will not flow through a locked joint, and that relaxation is practically impossible to achieve if you are holding tension in your joints. The best way to determine the proper amount of knee bend is to first lock the knees. Then slowly unlock them until the feeling of tension behind the knee disappears. Usually this is a matter of moving the knee forward perhaps 1 inch.

The pelvic girdle should be tilted slightly upward and forward, in order to straighten out the lower spine and keep the buttocks from protruding. This helps maintain an even balance and allows the energy to flow throughout the pelvic area.

The chest should be slightly "closed"—that is, don't puff out your chest like a soldier at attention; rather, bring the shoulder blades forward slightly. This closing of the shoulders is almost imperceptible, so don't force it. Again, the idea is to allow the Qi to flow unimpeded.

Speaking of shoulders, let them drop down and relax them completely. Each little bit of tension that you hold in the shoulders is transmitted throughout the arms and upper chest area, so make sure you relax. The elbows should be slightly bent, the wrists loose, and even the fingers should show a slight curl inward. All of these points of attention are again designed to both relax you and to open up the energy channels.

The head should be lifted up and supported as if a string were pulling upward on the very crown of your head. This further strengthens and straightens the spine, and ensures good posture and alignment. Tuck the chin in slightly, as most people have a tendency to lift their chins along with their heads. The end result of this alignment procedure should be that your gaze is level and calm, with a feeling that your spine is totally at ease and that your upper-body weight is flowing downward through your legs into the ground.

Finally, remember to keep the tongue gently touching on the upper palette of the mouth, just behind the front teeth. The most important reason for this unusual tongue placement is again related to energy flow—it bridges two of the main energy channels and allows the Qi to flow in a circuit throughout the body. Without the tongue in this position, the energy flows up the spine, over the head, and then comes to a halt—it does not continue it's journey back down the front of the body and back to the spine.

Remember also periodically during these exercises to stop and check your alignment and posture. In time, with repeated checking and conscientious practice, these alignment principles will become second nature.

Basic Stepping Exercises

Cat Stepping

Time to brush off that old cat and start stepping out again! Let's review what is involved in this unique stepping exercise.

The ability to visualize a clock face, the center upon which you are standing, is a great help in determining which direction to step. Failing this ability, pick out two reference points in your practice environment, such that they are at approximately 45 degrees to your right and left. If you are indoors, perhaps you can choose a lamp and a window as your reference points. Outdoors? That elm tree and the corner of the fence might do nicely.

From a neutral standing position, with your weight evenly distributed between both feet, slowly shift your weight to the left leg so that 70 percent of your body weight settles on the left side. Remember to accomplish this by bending the left knee slightly forward and lining your body up over the left leg. Now pull the right foot in toward your left foot, keeping it light and perhaps balancing on your right toes. With a smooth circular clockwise motion, and keeping your weight back on the left leg, sweep the right foot outward and slightly forward, such that the foot lands on its heel at the 2 o'clock position, perhaps 14 to 16 inches away from your left foot. The right toes should be pointing to 2 o'clock, and the right heel should point back at the left heel [Photo 75]. At this point, shift your body weight forward so that 70 percent is centered over your bent right leg. Make sure to keep the left foot flat on the ground and your back straight [Photo 76].

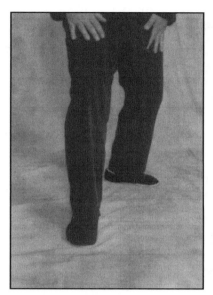

Photo 75.

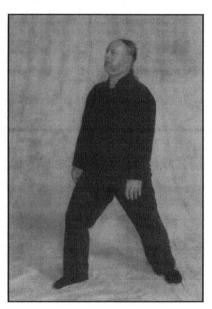

Photo 76.

If all went well, you should be facing 2 o'clock, with your weight shifted forward to your right leg, and your left foot behind you facing 12 o'clock. This is called a Bow Stance, because in this position you look like a bent bow, the right leg being the bow and the left leg being the drawn bowstring.

Now for the left leg. Shift all of your weight forward onto the bent right leg, bring the left foot up on its toes directly next to the right foot, and sweep the left foot out and around in a counterclockwise direction, landing on the left heel and with the left toes facing 10 o'clock. Once again, the step should be outward and slightly forward. Shift the weight forward onto the left leg approximately 70 percent, dropping the left foot flat and remembering to keep the right foot (facing 2 o'clock) flat also [Photo 77]. At this point, if you were to pull the left foot straight back toe-to-heel [Photo 78], the left heel would meet the right heel, and you would look somewhat like Charlie Chaplin!

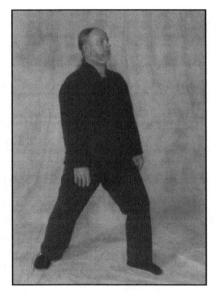

Photo 77.

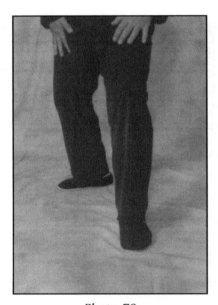

Photo 78.

Now continue this stepping movement, right side, left side, right side...aim for a balanced flow of movement, correct foot placement, and correct body alignment. Don't hold your breath! Just breathe slowly and naturally. Congratulations! You're doing T'ai Chi.

Basic T'ai Chi Hand Motions

Now we will see why I introduced Qigong before T'ai Chi. All of T'ai Chi's hand motions are identical to Qigong movements, with focus being placed on relaxed shoulders, bent elbows, soft wrist positioning, and relaxed and slightly curled fingers.

Arm Wave: Horizontal (Ward Off)

This exercise will prepare you for the T'ai Chi position known as Ward Off. Remember that T'ai Chi is by nature a martial art, and each of the positions has a martial meaning behind it. Ward Off is no different: it is used for pushing away your opponent with the back of your forearm.

Put your right hand in front of your body at chest level, slightly extended outward so that your elbow is slightly lower than your wrist. The shoulder should be

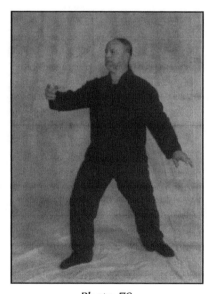

Photo 79.

relaxed and the wrist loose. The fingers point forward easily [Photo 79]. Now move the entire arm back and forth in front of you, flexing the wrist as you do so. Make believe you are stirring a big pot of soup with your hand—right to left and left to right. Make sure you lead with your wrist—the fingers trail behind the motion. So this means that when you go left to right, the fingers are pointing slightly left. When you go right to left, the fingers are pointing slightly backward to the right. This method of leading all hand movements with the wrists is basic to T'ai Chi movement. Continue the movement, again trying to achieve a smooth, flowing rhythm to the exercise. Remember to breathe!

Repeat this exercise with the left hand, again noting all of the proper alignment and movement principles.

Holding and Turning the Ball

Make believe you are holding a beach ball, about 12 inches in diameter, between both hands. You are holding the sides of the ball, so your palms face each other and the hands are slightly cupped or rounded. Hold the ball in front of your chest, about a foot away. Remember to relax the shoulders and elbows.

Now start to move the ball from the center to the right side of your body, turning your waist and hips but keeping your feet flat and parallel. As you do this, rotate the ball so that it goes through a quarter-turn. When you get as far as you comfortably can on the right side, your right hand should be on top of the ball, palm facing down, and the left hand should be on the bottom, palm facing up [Photo 80].

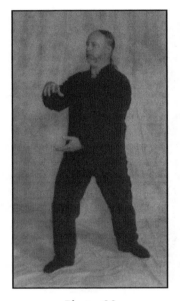

Photo 80.

Come back to the front of your body, once again rotating the ball through a quarter-turn and the hands now holding it at the sides. Now we'll go to the left side, turning the waist and hips and rotating the hands. When we get to the left side, the left hand should be on top of the ball, and the right hand on the bottom. Return to front and center.

Repeat the side-to-side motion, constantly turning the ball around its center and coordinating the movements. Don't feel bad if you can't get the hang of this right away. Just keep practicing and thinking, and you'll get it soon enough. This is the Holding the Ball posture in T'ai Chi, and is used for both flowing energy into the hands and striking your opponent with either hands or fists.

Pushing With Both Hands

Stand in a basic starting position. Bring both arms back, tucking your elbows into the sides of your body, and lift your fingers upward to point at the ceiling (or as close as possible). This is the preparation position for Pushing With Both Hands.

Now turn your upper body at the waist to the right side and push forward with both palms, keeping the fingers pointing upward. Imagine you are pushing a refrigerator. Keep your elbows slightly bent, even at the conclusion of the push, and remember to keep your body upright and balanced. Now bring the hands back toward the body, tucking the elbows once again against the ribs. Turn the body to the left, and repeat the push in that direction. Draw back to center, and repeat on both sides alternately.

The martial meaning of this movement is, of course, pushing your opponent away from you while maintaining your balance and not overextending your body.

Combining the Hands and Feet

Now for the toughest part—combining the foot and hand motions into one unified, graceful whole. When I say that it is the toughest part, don't run away; we'll go about this slowly and logically, and you'll soon be moving in a smooth, coordinated fashion. But don't worry about being "graceful" at this point. It's enough to understand and practice the movements themselves; over time, your movements will be flowing like a T'ai Chi Master!

First we'll practice the **Ward Off** movement that we learned in the previous section with the Cat Stepping exercise. This is a basic exercise in T'ai Chi, so when you master this exercise, you can truly say that you are a T'ai Chi player!

Begin in a basic starting position. By now, this should be a natural position for you, so you should be able to assume it without much difficulty. Perform a Cat Step out to your right side, and as you do so, Ward Off with your right hand and arm. If done properly, this movement should result in you being in a Right Bow Stance, with 70 percent of your weight on the right leg. Your body should be upright and relaxed, and your right arm should be aligned over your right leg, with the fingers pointing to the 2 o'clock position, as if getting ready to shake someone's hand. Now drop the right arm down to your side, Cat Step out to the left (10 o'clock position), and Ward Off with your left arm and hand. This will finish with your being in a Left Bow Stance and your left arm over your left leg, with the fingers pointing toward 10 o'clock. Drop the left arm. Repeat alternately on both sides.

One way to make this movement smoother is to "coil" your arm before Warding Off. To do this, cross your right arm over your chest, with the fingers pointing to the left, and execute a right Cat Step [Photo 81]. As you shift your weight onto the right leg, unwind or uncoil the right arm and allow it to smoothly arc into its finished position over the right leg. Drop the arm down, coil the left arm over the body, Cat Step to the left, and as you shift your weight onto the left leg, uncoil the arm into its final Ward Off position over the left leg. The resulting movements will be Step–Ward Off–Drop Arm, Step–Ward Off–Drop Arm. It becomes a type of dance, a coordination and balance exercise.

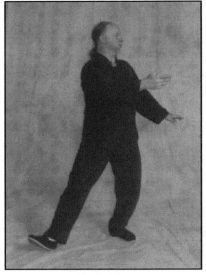

Photo 81.

Now let's try the **Holding the Ball** exercise with Cat Stepping. Probably the best way to start this one is to start doing the Hold the Ball exercise by itself, and add in the Cat Step at the appropriate moment. So, let's start Holding the Ball, beginning in the front of the body and progressing from center to right side, from right side back to center, and then to the left side. Get into the flow of it before you think about stepping.

When you are ready to step, bring the ball over to the left side of your body, left hand on top. Now perform a Cat Step out to the right side (2 o'clock position) while turning both your body and the ball. If done properly, you should end up in a Right Bow Stance holding a ball over your right leg, with your right hand on top of the ball. Now step out to the left (10 o'clock position), turning the ball over so that the left hand is on top and the ball is lined up over your left leg. Continue the movements, stepping and turning to both sides alternately.

Finally, let's try the **Pushing With Both Hands** movement with Cat Stepping.

Draw the hands into your body, tucking the elbows into your ribs, and Cat Step out to the right position. As your weight shifts forward, push out with both hands over your right leg. Make sure not to push so far that your back bends and your bottom juts out—your hands should push no further than your right foot. Remember that at this point, your rear foot is flat and your back is straight. Now, as you begin to bring your left foot up next to your right foot, draw the hands into the body again. Step to the left, and push over the left leg.

These are the basic T'ai Chi exercises that you can practice on your own in order to improve your coordination, balance, posture, and breathing. Breathing? Oops, we haven't really talked about breathing yet—I hope you haven't been holding your breath all this time!

Breathing Techniques for T'ai Chi Exercises

Breathing techniques for T'ai Chi are the same as they are for Qigong: you are trying to breathe diaphragmatically, without holding or forcing the breath. One way to remember the proper breathing is to think of the martial meaning of the movements. So, when you are Warding Off, or pushing someone away, you are exerting yourself and need to exhale. When you are beginning to step and are drawing your feet together, or are coiling your arm across your body, you are in a defensive mode, so you would then inhale.

Or think of lifting a heavy bag of groceries out of your car's trunk. Before you lift the bag, you get your hands into position underneath it, place your feet directly under your body, and inhale. Then when you actually start lifting, you exhale, straightening up your back and bringing the bag of groceries close to your body to maintain your center of gravity. If you were to reverse this breathing cycle, you would find that you are not as comfortable with the weight being lifted, or that you could not lift it at all. This follows the basic breathing principles of weight lifting: you inhale before you put forth your effort, and then exhale as you lift. The exhale tightens your stomach muscles and, in T'ai Chi at least, allows the Qi to flow through the body, aiding the lifting process.

Remember to keep a little reserve in your breathing. Don't force all of the air out of your lungs when you exhale; rather, keep 10 percent or so in reserve. Do the same when you inhale; don't inhale to the bursting point, but leave a little space left over. This keeps the body from straining and tensing up, a core principle of T'ai Chi. Not that we hold our breath in T'ai Chi (you should NEVER hold it) but it has been proven that you can hold your breath longer if you follow this rule than if you go for 100-percent capacity.

So whether you are Warding Off, Holding a Ball, or Pushing With Both Hands, you should exhale on the actual application or performance of the move, and inhale during the transitions or "in-between" times.

Chapter 8

We All Stand Up, We All Sit Down

Seated Adaptations of T'ai Chi and Qigong

Tradeoffs

While the wonders of T'ai Chi are accessible to everyone, no matter their age or physical condition, there are times when you need to modify the movements and postures in order to be able to effectively perform them. This chapter will outline the pros and cons of such modifications, along with step-by-step instructions for the seated movements.

Before we begin, let me clarify that seated T'ai Chi and Qigong are in no way inferior to the standing versions—merely different. Of course, you won't gain the balance you normally would in a standing version, nor will you experience the same type of energy flow patterns. But you can still breathe diaphragmatically, still work the arms, shoulders, wrists, and even, to an extent, the waist. You still reap the benefits of energy flow through the upper body and arms and, to a limited degree, the legs.

A basic sitting position involves the feet being placed flat on the floor. If you have short legs or a large chair, try to find a comfortable, yet supportive and firm chair to sit in. Dangling legs does not good T'ai Chi make! The ideal chair would be a wooden dining table–type chair, with no arms and a fairly straight back. Your back should be straight (again, within your personal limitations). The Chinese have a saying: The back of a chair is only for hanging your coat. If your back falls into the contours of the chair, in most instances, you'll be misaligned. The hands will be returning to a neutral position after most of the exercises. In the standing versions, we let our arms fall to our sides. But in seated position, you can simply let the hands rest on the knees or thighs. All of the breathing techniques, head support mechanics, and shoulder relaxation methods apply to seated T'ai Chi.

Basic Qigong Exercises

18-Movement Qigong Form

1. Origin: Lift arms to chest level, and then return hands to the knees.

2. Opening the Chest: Same as standing version except the hands return to the knees.

3. Painting the Rainbow: Here we need to make a slightly different type of adjustment. Because in the standing version we turn our feet, hips, and waist in the direction we are "painting," we need to try to duplicate that as much as possible. After your opening moves, you should be sitting upright with your arms out to your sides, palms up. When you paint with one or the other hand, turn your waist in the direction of the painting stroke as much as possible, without straining. Then simply let the hands return to your lap, and start over on the opposite side.

4. Parting the Clouds: Same as standing except, when the hands come down to your sides, bring them inward and over your lap. Remember to cross the wrists at the beginning of each repetition.

5. Whirling Arms on Horseback: Here you need to be careful not to tilt or tip in your chair. In the standing version, we shift our weight from side to side. In seated version, there's no need to shift weight; just perform the hand motions.

6. Rowing on the Lake: Same as standing. You will find, though, that if your chair has armrests, this movement can be rather difficult. This is why I recommended a dining room chair with no arms.

7. Holding a Ball at Shoulder Level: Hopefully your arm can reach at least a little ways behind the chair. If not, don't worry about it.

8. Gazing at the Moon Over the Shoulder: Same as standing version except, of course, the hands glide over your lap instead of hanging all the way down in front of you.

9. Press Palms Across the Body: Same as standing version.

10. Wave Hands Like Clouds: Lower hand passes over the lap.

11. Scoop the Sea and Look to the Sky: Lean forward as far as comfortable (without falling out of the chair!), scoop the sea, then raise yourself back up and lean into the back of the chair to look up into the sky (don't tilt the chair over backwards!).

12. Set the Waves Rolling: Same as standing without shifting the weight back and forth.

13. Dove Spreads Wings: Same as standing without the weight shift.

14. Punching From a Horseback Riding Stance: Same as standing; try placing your feet farther apart on the floor, but keep them parallel.

15. Wild Goose In Flight: Same as standing, without the heel lifting.

16. Turning the Windmill: No weight shifting. Turn the waist as much as comfortable in time with the arm rotations, gliding the hands over the lap at the bottom of the rotation.

17. Marching In Place While Bouncing the Ball: Wow, this one is easy now! Lift one hand and opposite foot. You will probably only be able to lift the foot a few inches, but that's okay.

18. Closing: Same as standing version.

There. That wasn't so bad, now, was it? Now let's try the Eight Pieces of Brocade in seated style.

Eight Pieces of Brocade Qigong Form

1. Double Hands Hold Up the Heavens: Same as standing version, except the hands come down to the lap at the end of the movement.

2. Aim the Bow and Shoot the Arrow: Same as standing version except, of course, no weight shifting from side to side. Do try to turn your waist as much as possible, however.

3. Alternately Supporting Heaven and Earth: Instead of keeping hands aligned on your centerline, they will float down gently to your sides.

4. Five Weaknesses and Seven Injuries Disappear: Same as standing version.

5. Sway the Head and Swing the Tail: Here again, we have a challenge. We need to lean over the sides of the chair as much as is comfortable, without falling. Please be very careful when you do this. Remember to keep your hands placed palm down on your thighs.

6. Lift and Touch Toes: Another challenging one. Reaching up isn't any different, but touching the toes—hmm, that's tough! Do the best you can—if you start to get dizzy, stop immediately.

7. Screw the Fists With Fiery Eyes: Same as standing. Try spreading the legs apart a little more to resemble a horseback riding position.

8. Feet and Head Lifted: Just lift the heels—no balance problems here.

And there you have it: the seated Qigong methods. Not all that different from the standing. One note here: There is a separate Seated Eight Pieces of Brocade

Qigong Form that I have not included here. Perhaps if there's enough interest in it, we can include it in the next book!

Basic T'ai Chi Hand Motions: Seated

With the seated T'ai Chi variations, let me just say this: This will *not* be "true" T'ai Chi, at least not the type that the Masters all perform in China. You won't have the same balance training, you won't feel your legs rooting into the ground during a push, and you won't be able to work those leg muscles and knee joints very much.

So what? You're still exercising, still moving, and hopefully, still breathing! With that quick introduction, let's try the exercises.

Ward Off

Seated Ward Off can be accomplished quite simply. Your seated position is the same as for the Seated Qigong exercises: straight back, lifted head, feet firmly planted. Lift the right arm up in front of you, with the hand at chest level, elbow slightly lower than wrist, shoulder relaxed, and fingers pointing forward with the thumb on top. Now turn your waist slightly to the right and allow the arm to follow the movement as far to the right as comfortable. Then turn the waist to the left and let the arm follow to the left side. Remember, as in the standing version of Ward Off, let the wrist be loose and let it lead the movement. The fingers should always trail behind the wrist during Ward Off.

Holding and Turning the Ball

Once again, ensure that your posture and alignment is correct while you are sitting. Keep that head up! Begin by holding the imaginary ball in front of your chest, elbows down, wrists bent, and shoulders relaxed. Make the ball about one foot or so in diameter.

Turn your waist to the right, simultaneously turning the ball so that your right hand finishes up on top of the ball, the left hand supporting the bottom. Now turn your waist to the front again, bring the hands on either side of the ball, and continue turning to the left, bringing the left hand on top, right hand on bottom. Continue for as long as comfortable, remembering not to tense up or allow the arms to tighten.

Pushing With Both Hands

Begin facing front. Draw the hands toward the chest, the elbows tucking into your sides against your ribs. Now turn the waist to the right, and push out gently with both hands. Don't reach too far—the elbows should still be slightly bent at the conclusion of the push.

Now draw the hands back to the chest as you simultaneously return your torso to the forward-facing position. Continue turning or coiling smoothly to the left, and push both hands in that direction.

Miscellaneous Seated T'ai Chi Exercises

Stretching One Arm Forward, Palm Up

Begin by holding an imaginary ball in front of your body at chest level, left hand on top (palm down), right hand on the bottom (palm up). Extend your right hand palm up in front of you as you drop the left hand and extend it down and behind you, palm down.

As you stretch the right hand forward and the left hand backward, stretch the upper body forward and turn it slightly to the right so that you face the direction that the right hand is stretching toward.

Turn the upper body back to a vertical, centered position and turn the right hand palm downward and the left hand palm up. Bring the arms together to hold the ball, this time with the right hand on top (palm down) and the left hand on the bottom (palm up).

Extend your left arm in front of you, palm up, and press your right hand down and behind you, palm down. Turn the upper body slightly to the left and incline forward.

Repeat several times on each side.

Lowering the Spine

Sitting in a chair that has armrests (wheelchair or regular chair), place your feet flat on the floor or on the footrests (with the wheels locked). Place your hands on the armrests.

Push your body upward (that is, off the chair) with both your hands and your feet, and then slowly let yourself back down. Use your legs as much as possible to lift and lower your body in this exercise.

The motions of this exercise are intended to strengthen the legs, improve the circulation throughout the body, and open the joints through which the circulation flows to and from the legs. This exercise can also begin to increase the flexibility of the spine.

White Crane Spreads Wings

This exercise, taken from the standing T'ai Chi form, is wonderful for increasing the range of motion of your shoulders, as well as working to eliminate pain from arthritis and rotator cuff injury.

Begin once again in seated position. Hold the ball in front of your body, left hand on top, palm down, and the right hand on the bottom, palm up.

Let the ball begin to shrink, such that your palms begin to approach each other. Now let the hands glide gracefully past each other without touching, the left hand continuing downward to your left side, the right hand stretching upward on the right side. At the completion of this move, your torso should be facing forward, your left arm down at your left side (slightly away from the chair) with the palm facing backwards and the fingers pointing down. Your right hand should be stretching upward at your right side, fingers pointing upward and palm facing forward.

Now reverse the hand motions, lifting the left hand up and allowing the right hand to drop. The left will rise in front of your body, palm up, while the right descends palm down. The hands will begin coming together as if holding the ball again, this time with the right hand on top. Continue the motion, letting the ball shrink and allowing the hands to pass by each other as they move to their new positions—the left hand reaching and pointing to the sky, palm forward, and the right hand reaching and pointing to the earth, palm backward.

Continue this movement, repeating several times on each side.

High Pat on Horse

This one is fun! Imagine that there's a large horse in front of you (how he got there is *your* problem!). You want to pat the horse's head, because he seems like a friendly beast.

Begin in the standard seated position, with both hands held at your sides at waist level, palms up. Now lift and extend the right hand forward and upward at a 45-degree angle, pushing with the palm and pointing the fingers upward. That's the patting hand. Keep the left hand palm up at your left side for now (perhaps that's the hand with the sugar cube!).

Now we'll switch hands. As you draw your right hand back into the side of your body, simultaneously turning it palm up, lift and extend the left hand in the same fashion as you did the right: fingers pointing up and pushing with the palm at a 45-degree angle.

Repeat several times on each side. This exercise works the shoulders, elbows, and wrists. It also helps increase your coordination (which, you're probably realizing by now, happens with all of these exercises).

Part III

Living in the Future

Chapter 9

Swimming in Serenity

Meditation Exercises

The Concept of Meditation

Meditation is the art of learning to quiet your mind so that the constant internal dialogue is turned off, at least for a few minutes a day, and you can enjoy a feeling of profound peace and happiness. It can be performed in many different ways—visualization, guided visualization, breath control, breath counting, problem-solving meditation for when you can't come up with the answers you need, and relaxation meditations for when you're stressed. Meditation can answer some very big questions that we all have: Why am I here? Where am I going? Who am I?

Why You Need to Meditate

Are you ever bothered by negative emotions—anger, fear, jealousy? Depressed, bored, or restless? Has life lost its meaning for you? If you never experience any of these, then you probably don't need to meditate. But for the rest of us, it's a wonderful tool!

Basically, we hold the power of making ourselves happy or unhappy. Now, you might be saying, "Well, what about when other people do bad things to me? I can't help how I respond to their meanness," Yes, you can!

Most people have known others who always seem happy, no matter what terrible event is taking place in their lives. They've also known people who are constantly miserable, no matter how wealthy or lucky they are. Do outside circumstances rule these people? Nope—it's really all in their heads. It's how they perceive reality, not how reality really is. Now, I know this may seem kind of *Twilight Zone*-ish, but it's true.

We choose how we feel. No one else can do that for us. We can allow ourselves to be hurt by the actions of others, or we can learn to balance ourselves, learn who and what we really are, through meditation practice. In this way, we are building ourselves up, defending ourselves mentally and emotionally against the cold, cruel world.

A Life of Constant Stress

For many of us today, life is one fight-or-flight response after another. Our society has decided to go into warp speed, and thinks it needs instant gratification in order to live a full life, forgetting that often it is the journey, and not the destination, that is important.

So we are always priming ourselves for battle, whether it is with the government or the grocery clerk. We develop a mindset of "Oh, no, you don't" before the events even come into being. This is emotional baggage of the highest order. And much like real-life baggage, we can choose whether it is worth carrying, or if we should just put it down on the side of the road and leave it for someone else.

Why Don't We Meditate?

In my years of teaching meditation, I've heard probably most of the possible responses to this question. It is easy to justify a non-action, but to actually have the gumption to get up and do something, well, that's a different story.

Some of the excuses I've been given as to why meditation would not be appropriate or possible include:

- It takes too long to learn.
- I could never relax that much.
- I'm not a "New Age"-type.
- Lots of people seem to start meditation classes, but don't stick with it. If meditation is so good, why does this happen?
- It works for some people, but not for me.
- I don't have the willpower to stick to it.
- People are sheep—they'll try anything.
- I don't have time to meditate. I'm too busy.
- I'm not a Communist—I don't do that kind of stuff.

Let me address a few of these to set your mind at rest about what meditation is and what it is not.

"It takes too long to learn."

No, it doesn't. I can teach you to meditate in about an hour. The rest is up to you. Understanding, practice, experimentation—that's all something that *you* have to want to do. But learning the basics, enough to actually begin meditating, goes by rather quickly.

"I could never relax that much."

"It only works for certain people."

Not true. Everyone can learn to relax; some just have a more arduous trail to success in front of them. The folks who claim these statements are usually afraid of trying new things and are afraid of change.

"People don't stick with it."

People these days are notoriously fickle when it comes to learning a new art or ability. They may start the classes with wonderful intent, thinking about all the wonderful things they've heard about meditation. When they actually are in class, however, and are asked to begin meditating, then it becomes "put up or shut up" time. Many people freeze at this point. The IDEA of meditation is wonderful. The REALITY and PRACTICE takes discipline, effort, and intent.

Don't worry about what other people do—do what *you* want to do.

"I don't have time to meditate."

Do you have time to go quietly insane? Because that's what might happen if you continue to live your life on the edge, running from one appointment to the next, never taking time to smell the roses.

Funny thing about meditation. When you perform it early in the morning, your day just seems to go by smoother, with fewer problems. It almost seems that time has slowed down, or expanded to meet your needs. Your mindset, established through the meditation, has allowed you to face life head-on and not flinch in the process.

How Is Meditation Related to T'ai Chi and Qigong?

Lately, Westerners have been hearing more and more about experimenting with visualization for improving one's physical performance and mental attitude. Books on using visualization for improving one's success in business and the power of imagery in healing are also gaining acceptance in our present-day society. T'ai Chi has been using imagery since T'ai Chi began around 1200 A.D. When practicing T'ai Chi, the colorful descriptions used for different passages, such as "wave hands in clouds" or "crane spreads wings" conjure mental images that influence the quality of the movement. Because the practice of T'ai Chi is precise and also imaginative, both hemispheres of the brain are drawn into play. The use of the right and left brain draws out the most potential in an individual. A relaxing, yet strengthening technique such as T'ai Chi develops the whole person, in mind, body, and spirit. It is not something that can only be talked about in theory, but needs to be experienced.

Even the learning of T'ai Chi and Qigong exercises can be a meditation. When we learn a new movement in class (or from this book), we first attempt to understand it with our rational, logical mind. We follow that initial understanding by physically trying the movement, then thinking some more, practicing some more, and so on. When you are so involved in this process that, hours later, you look at the clock and see that it's much later than you thought—you're meditating. You were in a different world for a while, devoting your concentration exclusively to T'ai Chi. You didn't worry about the bills, or the grandchildren, or taxes—you were living in the moment, enjoying your learning experience. That's meditation.

Another link to T'ai Chi is found in the concept of Qi itself. Certain meditations use a visualization of energy (Qi) flowing through the body in a prescribed manner. This increases your concentration and focus, once again taking you "outside of yourself." T'ai Chi and Qigong, of course, use the Qi to produce power and healing in the body.

At the higher levels of T'ai Chi practice, it is said that the practitioner is performing "moving meditation." This simply means that the T'ai Chi player is going beyond the physical aspects of the form, and is drawing in her concentration, thinking about guiding the energy down to her legs and arms. It is said that "the mind leads the Qi; the Qi leads the body." Therefore, you have as an end result the mind leading the body.

Basic Styles of Meditation

There are several different ways of classifying meditation that we will explore in this section. You can differentiate them according to their place of origin. Hence, you can study Western, Eastern, Buddhist, Taoist, Shinto, Hindu, Indian, Chinese, Christian, and so on.

You can also categorize them by name or type: visualization, Transcendental Meditation (TM), breath counting, problem solving, spiritual advancement, and physical healing.

Western meditation methods tend to be "newer" styles—that is, because we are such a relatively young country, we don't have the long history of experimentation with meditation that, say, the Hindus have. We have had some big hits—Transcendental Meditation, or TM, was quite popular in the 1960s and 70s. But most of the Western methods are modifications or adaptations of older, Eastern methods.

Eastern methods encompass many schools of practice—Buddhist, Taoist, Shinto, and Hindu are among the main ones. Their styles often pose a problem for Western practitioners: the basic philosophies of life, how we view the universe and ourselves, may be quite different than the Eastern viewpoint. So we may have difficulty absorbing some of the core concepts. In the meditation techniques I give in this book, I try to make them easy and understandable in light of our culture.

Indian and Hindu methods are perhaps some of the oldest ones in existence. Their version of guiding the energy, or prana, through the body is roughly equivalent to the Chinese concept of Qi flow. They concern themselves with chakras, where the Chinese model is meridians and channels. But the underlying theory—that there is an innate energy source in the human body that can be used for health and harmony—is the same.

Buddhist methods often use meditation to elevate spirituality and rid the meditator of earthly attachments. There are dozens of styles of Buddhism, but they all share the common thread of performing meditation as a central exercise to refine the mind and spirit. Zen Buddhism, sort of a cross between Buddhism and Taoism (see Chapter 11) uses koans, or riddles, that cannot be solved by logic or intellect, but must be meditated upon theoretically until enlightenment occurs.

Taoist methods of meditation borrow from the other styles and add their own unique flavor. The core concepts of Taoist meditation are to achieve a balance in the mind, body, and spirit through such exercises as observing the breath and contemplating one's role in the universe, or Tao. T'ai Chi is also a Taoist method of meditation, one in which you are moving while meditating upon the energy flow in the body.

Posture and Breathing

A quick review of the basic postural and mechanical requirements of meditation is in order at this point, before we proceed to the actual meditation exercises.

Here's a pleasant surprise for you: You already know the proper physical techniques. We have learned and practiced them throughout our T'ai Chi and Qigong exercises. Just to summarize, here they are again:

- Whether sitting or standing in meditation, your head should be lifted slightly upward, as if being pulled up by a string.

- The tip of your tongue should be lightly touching the upper palate, just behind the upper incisors.

ᔡ Shoulders and arms should be relaxed. If you are standing, the hands should fall comfortably to your sides. If sitting, there are a few options for hand placement. You can adopt a Western method and just let the hands rest on your thighs or knees, palms down. If you go with Eastern methods, the palms are usually held facing up in your lap, the fingertips almost but not quite touching. A variation of this pose is to lay the back of one hand in the palm of the other, the tips of the thumbs touching lightly. This is said to ensure a continuous energy pathway, and is perhaps one of the most commonly seen positions when meditation is practiced.

Breathing techniques are also similar to the T'ai Chi and Qigong exercises. Especially in a seated meditation, diaphragmatic breathing is the preferred method. Remember to expand the lower abdomen, and then the chest, as you inhale; contract first the lower abdomen, and then the chest, as you exhale. The idea is to utilize the diaphragm located below the lungs to ensure a deep, relaxed breath. The breath will be playing yet another role in our meditations here—we will be observing the breathing cycle as a means of relaxing and focusing.

Meditation Exercises

In this section, we will learn eight different meditation techniques, two each from four different categories of meditation. The categories used here will be breath counting, visualization, relaxation, and healing. Once again, realize that there are dozens of categories of meditation, and that this section is meant to be only a sampler of the available techniques. If you wish to explore these methods in more depth, New Page Books has many meditation titles available.

Breath Counting

Breath counting is simply a method of meditation in which you count the number of breaths you are taking. There are several variations that you can employ in this exercise:

ᔡ Count the inhale and exhale as one breath.

ᔡ Count separate inhales and exhales.

ᔡ Count the breaths until you lose count.

ഔ Count up only to a small number, say three or four. (This is the method we will explore here.) The purpose of keeping the count low is to en-sure that you don't begin to fixate on the count itself, but rather to keep your mind on the act of breathing. We don't want to make medita-tion a competitive sport, and this often happens with the counting-style meditations—"I got to 27 last time. Maybe I can get to 30 today!" That's not what meditation is all about; it's about relaxing and focusing.

To perform the breath-counting meditation, sit in a comfortable chair with your feet flat on the ground, your back fairly straight, and your head upright. Your hands can be placed in any of the previously mentioned positions: on your knees, in your lap, in your lap with palms up, or in your lap with palms nested together and the thumbs lightly touching.

Now, breathe. Breathe in through the nose. (We will use nose breathing through-out all of these meditation exercises. Unless you have a deviated septum, asthma, etc., this is the preferred method. If you need to, breathe through the mouth. It won't be the end of the world, and you will still gain the benefits of the meditation). Your eyes can remain open, you can close them completely or, as the Taoist monks often do, you can close them halfway. This eliminates the visual distractions around you, but ensures that you don't fall asleep. (This was a common difficulty, espe-cially among the monks, whose day would often begin before sunrise and continue through until late evening. In fact, it is said that one monk would walk around the temple with a "Stick of Enlightenment": when he came upon another monk who had fallen asleep during meditation, he would soundly whack him with the stick. I don't recommend this practice to my students!)

Remember that if you are breathing diaphragmatically, your breaths will be deeper and more relaxed, and you will bring a fresh supply of oxygen to the very bottom of your lungs. Your concentration at this point is simply to breathe, slowly and evenly. Never hold your breath, at least not in these beginning exercises—breath-holding is an advanced technique, which can be troublesome for those with high blood pressure or heart problems.

It may take a few minutes, but gradually, you should find yourself relaxing some-what more than usual. Your body will begin to feel heavy, and you will feel the day's tensions draining from your body. Let this feeling of peace wash over and through you like a cleansing spring rain, removing all of your troubles and con-cerns. Enjoy this feeling for as long as you like—we're not in any hurry!

Once you have enjoyed this newfound feeling of stress release, it's time to be-gin counting your breaths. This will do several things: It will increase your powers of concentration and focus; it will ensure that your mind doesn't wander; and it will provide a framework, or purpose, to the meditation. Often, when the word *meditation* is brought up in casual conversation, there is usually one person who says, "I could never meditate—I can't think of nothing!" In reality, it would be extremely difficult, if not impossible, to "think of nothing." That is not the purpose of meditation, as you are beginning to find out.

Back to the breath counting. Start at the beginning of one of your inhales. Breathe in, exhale, and think to yourself (don't say it out loud) "One." Repeat the inhale/exhale cycle, and think "Two." Repeat, and think "Three." Start the next cycle, and begin again at "One." Continue this breathing and counting routine for as long as you like.

You are now meditating! Of course, even with this simple meditation, there are a few things to be on the lookout for. First and foremost, don't think about anything but your breathing as you do this exercise. That will destroy all of the benefits of the meditation. Just enjoy the counting process, and don't get "hung up" on the counting. Also, don't worry during the exercise if you are "doing it right." Believe me, if you are sitting, breathing, and counting, you're doing it properly. If you lose track of what number you are on, no problem—just start over at "One."

Over time, as you practice this meditation (hopefully on a daily basis), you will be able to start the exercise easier, without all of the fuss of preparation involved in these first attempts. You will be able to just sit down, breathe, and count. It's a wonderful, quick, and relaxing way of getting rid of the day's troubles, as well as a good way to start your day.

Another breath-counting meditation is similar to this one, but we will be counting backwards. This is somewhat akin to the methods used in hypnosis, where the client counts backwards from 100, and by the time he or she reaches the lower numbers, they are fully hypnotized. Now, don't worry, I'm not going to hypnotize you here!

Start the breathing method used in the first meditation, making sure you are physically comfortable in your chair. Enjoy once again the simple pleasure of breathing fully and slowly. Feel yourself relaxing throughout your entire body.

Now, on the next inhale, say to yourself, "Ten." Continue to breathe slowly..."Nine" on the next inhale...feel yourself almost sinking down to the ground..."Eight"...you are fully relaxed at this point...and so on, all the way back to "One." But what happens when you get to "One"? Do you use negative numbers? No, simply forget about the counting, and simply enjoy the process of breathing. At this point, you can actually move into the Breath-Watching meditation, which is the first visualization meditation we will try.

Visualization Meditations

Much has been written and claimed for visualizations. They are a way of directing our intent, or our will, in whichever direction we desire. It is said that to make something happen, you must *see* it happening in your mind. This is the main power of visualization. For our purposes, we might be more interested in the ability of visualization to hone our concentration and allow us to forget our troubles for a while.

In our first visualization meditation, **Breath Watching**, we will be doing just that: watching our breath. Sounds like watching paint dry, right? Trust me, it's a bit more beneficial to your health to watch your breath.

We begin by assuming the standard meditation position. By now, you should be getting a bit more comfortable in this position. If not, experiment—change the chair you use, change the position of your hands, close your eyes if they're open.

Now relax into your breathing. Breathe deeply and slowly, feeling the breath fill you up with lightness and health. Once you are settled in your breathing rhythm, you can start your visualization. What we will be doing at this point is imagining that we can see the air that we're breathing. Perhaps you can imagine that the air looks like a golden liquid, or a white vapor. My students have come up with all manner of ideas for what air "looks" like. The important thing here is that you are comfortable with the look.

As you continue your breathing, see the air around you in your chosen color and consistency. Now watch it as it enters your body through your nose as you inhale. It travels down to your lungs, and actually goes all the way down to your lower abdomen, to a point just below your navel. Now, of course, the air is not really going that far, unless you have leaky plumbing, but it's the visualization that is important here.

By the end of the inhale, you should have a full breath of air, and your attention is directed at your lower abdomen. Now for the exhale. As you begin to exhale, follow the breath as it leaves your abdomen, goes through your body to the base of your spine, follows the spine all the way up to your head, and then travels over the top of your head and back out your nose into the world. That was one cycle of breathing, a simple enough thing really, but your mind followed an imaginary pathway throughout your upper body. This ability to visualize is extremely important in meditation, as well as in energy healing, and even advanced T'ai Chi practice, where you are visualizing the flow of Qi throughout the body.

Continue the exercise, watching the next inhale travel down the front of your body, and then up your spine, over your head, and out your nose on the exhale.

Repeat as many times as possible, until you either get tired or bored. There's no use in forcing a meditation. Sometimes you just are not in the mood, and you can develop resentment for meditation if you attempt to do it during those times.

Our second visualization meditation will be called **Vacation**. The purpose will be to imagine yourself in your favorite vacation spot. It doesn't matter if you've never actually been there, as long as you can imagine it. What this meditation does first is to improve your thought and imagination processes, a benefit of special interest to us as we get older. We need to exercise the mind as well as the body to stay young. Secondly, this exercise is great for those times when you wish you could get away on a vacation, but for economic or practical reasons, cannot. It's like a miniature mind-vacation, and I guarantee that you'll return feeling refreshed.

By now, you know that you should relax into your starting position, releasing whatever physical tensions are present by first stretching or doing your T'ai Chi exercises. Once you are comfortably settled in, start concentrating on your breathing. Slow and easy does it. Spend a little while enjoying the breathing process and getting into that relaxed state.

At whichever point you wish, continuing the breathing uninterrupted, switch your attention to a little scene that you play in your mind. That scene is your favorite vacation spot, whether it is the beach, the mountains, the woods, or Las Vegas! *See* that place in as much detail as you can in your mind's eye. See the colors, smell the smells, hear the bustle of nature (or people) flowing around and through you. The idea here is to recreate that place as faithfully as possible.

Take as much time as you need in establishing the initial scene, and add as much detail as you are able. Once you've set the stage, explore it. Walk around, see things from different angles and heights, hear new sounds and smell new odors. Make it as real as if you were actually there. Enjoy your vacation!

Now, a word about returning to the "real" world. Often after a meditation, it can be difficult to return to the everyday world. You feel so good when you're meditating that you don't want to stop. But at some point, we *do* need to return. So, do it as gently as possible to minimize the shock. When you are ready to leave your vacation spot, visualize yourself returning to the place where you began the trip. The sounds are beginning to recede into the distance, you can't smell as many scents as you did before, and even the colors of the surrounding areas are beginning to fade. Slowly bring your concentration back to your breathing, perhaps watching the breath come down the front of the body and exit up the spine and out the nose. Take your time. Slowly open your eyes as you return fully to the here and now.

Refreshing, wasn't it?

Relaxation Meditations

Although all of the previously discussed meditations are relaxing, these next two are specifically designed to relax your body as well as your mind. The first one is the **Heavy Meditation**.

Start in your normal meditation position, and watch your breath for a few minutes. Gradually shift your attention away from your breath and into your body. Attempt to feel your body growing heavy in your chair. Feel your weight increasing as your shoulders drop downward and your feet are cemented in place on the floor. But don't let your head fall forward—keep it pulled upward by that invisible string.

As you inhale, you can feel yourself lighten a little bit and begin to feel as if you are floating upward. On the exhale, you once again feel the pull downward, as if you could not get out of your chair even if you tried. This is what true relaxation feels like—as if you are melting into the ground.

To come back from your meditation, switch your focus back to your breathing, watching it travel through your body. Slowly open your eyes and return to the here and now.

The second relaxation meditation is the **Stomach Softening** meditation. Assume your beginning position, and watch your breath for a few minutes. Then focus your attention on your stomach. Is there any tension there? Are you unconsciously holding it in? Let it go. Let it be loose.

Now place the palms of both hands gently over your stomach. As you inhale, the hands ride up with your stomach. As you exhale, they ride back down. This is a great way to practice diaphragmatic breathing, in addition to its use as a relaxation exercise. We often hold many of our tensions in our stomach; this meditation allows us to release those tensions and gain greater health in the process.

Unlike the previous meditation, this one does not require any visualization—just feel the hands rise and fall on the stomach. Finish up by bringing your attention back from the stomach to the breath, and from there back to your surroundings.

Healing Meditations

Pain—we've all experienced it. You can't get through life without it. But how we deal with pain is at least as important as searching for a way to get rid of it. These two final meditations are designed to recognize and deal with your pain, whether it is emotional, mental, or physical in nature. Be forewarned that these meditations can bring out some strong emotional reactions such as crying and sobbing. This is natural—it's the release of the pain that we're working toward. Just remember that this is a temporary pain—one that we invoke in order to eliminate the long-term pain.

The first exercise is called the **Compassion Meditation**. We will be taking a tour of our life through this meditation, starting at the earliest point of our youth that we can recall.

Assume your starting posture and watch your breath for a few minutes. Now remember back to the earliest point of your childhood that you can. See yourself, as you were, whether it was happy and carefree or sad and burdened. Give yourself a mental hug and send loving compassion to that little child.

Repeat this inspection and expression of compassion for yourself at the subsequent life stages of older child, puberty, young adult, all the way to your present self. At this last stage, give yourself an especially big hug (use your hands and arms if you like!), bathing yourself in love and compassion. For many of us, compassionate feelings for ourselves are secondary to our concern for others. But to heal ourselves, we need to love ourselves first.

The second healing meditation is called the **Softening Meditation**. Start in your usual position, observe your breath for a few minutes, and then pick out a minor pain that you have in your physical body. It can be a headache, some low-back pain, arthritis in the fingers—whatever you choose—but start with a minor one, not a major one.

Put your focus on the pain while you continue your deep, relaxed breathing. Try to envision what the pain looks like, not what it feels like. See it as perhaps a red area on your body, with little lightning bolts issuing from it. Just observe the pain; don't make judgments about it ("It's worse today than yesterday") or pity yourself. Use the pain as your meditational focus point. Imagine the pain beginning to soften as you watch it—the red color growing pale pink, the lightning bolts slowing and finally stopping. Incorporate some relaxation meditation techniques here—feel yourself growing heavy in your chair, switch back and forth from watching your breath to watching the pain.

This meditation will take some practice to use, but I think it's practice well worth the effort. If we can control or eliminate our pain by using our minds, the possibilities are endless.

Chapter 10

Paging Dr. Chi

T'ai Chi in the Rehabilitation Setting

Using T'ai Chi in Rehabilitation

The art of T'ai Chi has, for centuries, been used as a martial art, as a defense against opposing armies, and as a preventative exercise system. Only recently here in the West have we discovered another facet of T'ai Chi, that of rehabilitation.

Within the last 20 years there have been many studies made by medical professionals with the assistance of T'ai Chi instructors in the use of T'ai Chi movement principles in restoring nominal levels of health. In addition to the physical therapy provided by the movements themselves, a large part of the healing ability of T'ai Chi lies in the internal aspects of the art: the visualizations, imagery, and energy flow considerations. These internal aspects help bring forth a holistic, mind/body healing modality that can be used effectively in conjunction with Western medicine or, in some cases, by itself.

There are several ideas concerning exactly *how* T'ai Chi can effect these cures. One theory is that the physical movement itself is primarily responsible for healing; that the slow, gentle motions of the T'ai Chi form are merely a variant of existing physical therapy range-of-motion exercises performed every day in hospitals and rehab centers throughout the world. This perhaps is a simplification, because T'ai Chi can be, and is, so much more. Again, here in the West we have been trained to place our confidence in purely physical cures, disregarding the role that the mind plays in the healing equation. T'ai Chi makes no such mistake—it realizes that the body, without the control of the mind, is merely an empty vessel.

Another Western perspective is that Qi does not exist, because it cannot be found on X-rays or CAT scans. It is postulated that what actually happens is that the blood flow is improved through the T'ai Chi exercises, leading to a healing state for limited cases of incapacitation. This viewpoint also reduces T'ai Chi to some type of slow-motion physical therapy, refusing to acknowledge that our bodies are a complex web of interwoven physical parts and mental attitudes. Being a

Chinese modality, T'ai Chi borrows from Taoist thought and sees the entire person, not just a physical body, with its allied brain, emotions, thoughts, energy, and spirit. To divorce one from the other is to treat the symptoms, but not the root cause of the pain.

On the positive side, patient empowerment and self-care, as well as medical cost-reduction possibilities have a special potential to transform medicine as it is practiced in the Western world. However, the aspect of T'ai Chi that has greatest potential to restructure medicine, as we know it, is the amazing technique of "external" Qigong. In external Qigong, the practitioner or Qigong doctor does non-touch energy assessment of the patient and actually projects or conducts Qi, in a treatment mode, to the patient.

In assessment, rather than asking questions, taking pulses, observing the tongue, palpating reflexes, and ordering lab tests, the practitioner uses concentration, intuition, and reading of the Qi with off-the-body diagnostic scanning. In treatment, the practitioner actually projects the Qi to another to have a clinical effect. Both of these techniques seem impossible and fantastic. However, research is revealing that there may be authentic, explainable, and demonstrable natural laws and mechanisms in operation during these events. Therapeutic Touch, an assessing and healing technique that uses an "off the body" technique called "unruffling the field" has experienced a tremendous swell of interest in the nursing community. The research of developer Delores Krieger, RN, demonstrated that in-vivo hemoglobin values (an essential blood-quality component) were significantly affected by the administration of this energy-based technique.

An October 1986 article in the *Los Angeles Times* tells the story of the Beijing practice of Master Xun Yunkun who treats medical cases including terminal cancer and paralysis following stroke with Qi projection.

There is a tremendous wave of interest in this aspect of Qigong in the Western world and a number of very respectable research organizations are currently expending substantial budgets on Qigong-related projects. There is a tremendous amount of research attempting to explain this phenomenon. The American Foundation of Traditional Chinese Medicine, Dr. Zheng Rong, and Stanford physicist Professor William Tiller are doing a collaborative research project on bioluminescence and Qigong with a focus on satisfying the rational research model. In 1988, 128 research papers were presented at the First World Conference for the Academic Exchange of Medical Qigong that was sponsored by the China Medical Association, Chinese Ministry of Health, China Qigong Research Institutes, and the Beijing College of Traditional Chinese Medicine and was attended by representatives from 17 countries.

On one hand, it is wonderful that there may be Qigong doctors with such special abilities. It would be a shame, however, if we became so dependent upon their abilities that we ignored the benefits derived from self-applied Qigong techniques.

In my own practice, I have accepted clients who, having failed to make any noticeable progress in months of physical therapy, began to despair of ever regaining their former health. Through a progressive program of T'ai Chi exercises, occasionally combined with Chinese medicine and meditation practice, these clients soon regained use of limbs formerly frozen in place, became highly mobile after long periods of being restricted to wheelchairs, and improved such lifestyle staples as diet, nutrition, sleep patterns, and psychological outlooks on life.

I have been working as a T'ai Chi instructor in a local facility, the John Heinz Institute of Rehabilitative Medicine in Wilkes-Barre Township, Pennsylvania, for more than four years now, and the results for many of the students are amazing. Students, who after attending physical therapy sessions for long periods of time, often come to my classes after experiencing strokes, heart attacks, seizures, and various bodily injury. While their progress is due, in part, to the diligent work of dedicated therapy professionals, they have not usually had the mental or spiritual component of their injuries or illnesses addressed. This is one of the many uses of T'ai Chi in a rehabilitative setting—integrating Eastern and Western medicine.

One of my students has made what I would call a miraculous recovery. She came to one of my biannual seminars on T'ai Chi with advanced arthritis, extremely low energy levels, restricted range of motion, and a somewhat depressed outlook on life. You couldn't blame her—she was expecting to spend her life in a wheelchair. After attending the seminar, she signed up at my school and studied hard for three years. The result? Lots of energy, almost unbelievable range-of-motion improvement, arthritis that had just about disappeared, and a positive outlook on life. She is now teaching T'ai Chi to her own students and conveying the wonders of this rehabilitative art to many others.

Study at Emory University

Those of us with a regular T'ai Chi practice intrinsically understand its value for everything from physical fitness to spiritual fulfillment. In communicating our enthusiasm for T'ai Chi, what we often lack is the kind of hard evidence for T'ai Chi's value that can break through the wall of skepticism put up by many Westerners.

That's why a study sponsored by the National Institute on Aging (NIA) is so encouraging. As published in the May 3, 1995, issue of the *Journal of American Medical Association* (*JAMA*), T'ai Chi was the only exercise/activity to show a statistically significant decrease in the number of falls among the elderly study participants. The T'ai Chi practitioners recorded a 25 percent decrease in injuries from falls. Some of the other exercise modules showed increased falls, merely because the patients were moving more. In resistance or flexibility training, there's the tendency to go too far too fast. That's when people get hurt. The nature of T'ai Chi is helping people understand the value of moderation, which has always made it the safest of exercise.

More than 30 percent of people aged 65 or older experience at least one fall per year, and 15 percent of those falls result in serious injuries. Falls are the sixth largest cause of death among seniors and contribute to a general health decline even when they're not the direct cause of death. Falls are expensive. The last figures are from 1984—before the aging trend got into full swing, and before the recent inflation of medical costs. Even back in 1984, falls of senior citizens cost $3.7 billion a year.

Unlike anecdotal evidence that the skeptical can shrug off as Eastern mysticism, this study involved eight medical facilities, including some of the most esteemed names in Western medical science: Harvard, Yale, Centers for Disease Control, Washington University School of Medicine, and Emory University.

The slow pace so emphasized in T'ai Chi is alive and well in Western medical research. This groundbreaking study lasted 12 years, resulting in final publication of results in 1984. That's not a bad thing, per se. In fact, it highlights how *good* research is *careful* research that isn't hurried. By 1989, the NIA came together with the National Center for Nursing Research and the Centers for Disease Control to issue a Request for Applications. Of 42 proposals, eight were chosen and funded as of April 1990. The studies took place over the ensuing three years, concluding in March 1993. Since then, it's been a matter of follow-up—tracking the incidence of falls, data analysis, and peer review. Addressing the ongoing value of T'ai Chi training, the *JAMA* article notes, "It is encouraging that the reduction in risk persists...for a median time of 1.5 years."

The T'ai Chi component of the study took place at Emory University in Atlanta, Georgia, under the supervision of Dr. Steve Wolf from the Department of Rehabilitative Medicine. While the *JAMA* article did much to open doctors' eyes to T'ai Chi's benefits, it didn't go into detail about the T'ai Chi study. Wolf forged ahead with a more detailed report for the *Journal of the American Geriatric Society*. After some frustrating delays in the process, the report finally appeared in the May 1996 issue of the *Journal*. Emory is known for its open-minded approach to finding healthcare solutions. In a typically Taoist example of convergence, it so happened that T'ai Chi Master Tingsen Xu was a visiting professor of Biochemistry at Emory in 1990 when it came time to put this study together. Wolf said, "We worked with Xu to synthesize the 108 moves down to 10 that we felt from a physiotherapeutic and rehab perspective represented movements that often become compromised in folks as they get older—most notably trunk and body rotation and the ability to maintain a narrower base of support."

The Emory study compared T'ai Chi to the expensive, technologically advanced Chattecx Balance System of Chattanooga Corp. Chattecx uses an independently mounted balance platform for each foot. The subjects' feet are hooked to sensors, four on each foot—front left, front right, rear left, rear right. They view a cursor that represents their center of balance on a computer monitor. Subjects were told to keep their balance aligned perfectly and trained to improve their performance, kind of like an interactive video game for senior citizens. The premise relies on biofeedback; showing participants their actual center of balance is intended to help them better maintain that center of balance even when they're not hooked up to the machine. And it did work.

Wolf points out that the balance-platform participants could maintain their center of balance better than T'ai Chi students, but that this didn't help them outside the laboratory. "The notion of training people, especially older people, to maintain their center of mass within their base of support as the way to secure safety, is not necessarily correct," he stated. The world isn't a place where we stand with our feet parallel and try to orient ourselves to a computer screen. In the real world, we walk in poor light, encounter unfamiliar obstacles and traverse uneven ground. "You have to be placed in dynamic situations so you can develop strategies that will enable you to succeed in regaining your balance," said Wolf. In these real-world situations, T'ai Chi's renowned centering principles made the difference that no other exercise could match.

The Emory study looked at seven therapeutic benefits for T'ai Chi:

1. Continuous movement.

2. Small to large degrees of motion depending on the individual.

3. Flexed knees with distinct weight shifts between legs.

4. Straightening and extending head and trunk for less "flexed" posture. Attention developed to prevent leaning of trunk or protrusion of the sacrum.

5. Trunk and head rotates as a unit during circular movements that emphasize rotation. Eyes follow movement, promoting head and trunk rotation through eye centering and eye movements.

6. Asymmetrical and diagonal arm and leg movements promote arm swing and rotation around the waist axis.

7. Unilateral weight bearing with constant shifting to and from right and left legs to build strength for unilateral weight bearing and improve unilateral balance through knowledge of one's balance limitations and practice of movements within those limitations.

Compare these benefits with the list of conditions that all exercise programs for the elderly must address:

- Slowed movement.
- Reduced range of motion and strength.
- Increased flexed/stooped/posture.
- Reduced rotational movements.
- Limited arm swing.
- Decreased unilateral weight bearing.

This list of T'ai Chi's benefits is a virtual recipe for alleviating these common problems in the elderly. The most significant difference between T'ai Chi and other exercises is awareness. There's nothing special about the T'ai Chi movements in and of themselves. As any Master will confirm, if the moves are performed without concentration, T'ai Chi is merely exercise. But there is something very "present" about its emphasis on awareness. And according to the study, "training for balance may partly work not just because it increases the limits of stability and balance per se, but because the subject becomes aware of his or her limits of stability and allows compensation for the deficits."

The T'ai Chi moves in this study are a simplified selection from the first third of the yang style. This modified form begins, naturally enough, with Origin. The following nine moves from the study were:

1. Ward off Left.
2. Push Left.
3. Cloudy Hands.
4. Single Whip.
5. Ward off Left.
6. Brush Left Knee, Push Right.

7. Kick Right.

8. Kick Left.

9. Close.

Even with such a simple selection of yang moves, it's significant that Xu taught less than one move each week, despite meeting twice per week. Think how that compares to the more common goal of teaching two moves per week.

For impatient youth, two moves a week may be necessary to maintain student interest. But that needn't be the case. While everyone wants to feel that they're making progress, that progress can take shape in ways other than new moves. Xu was able to keep his students interested in the principles and the details by showing them the immediate benefit to their training. By emphasizing their growing awareness and centeredness, Xu showed his students a greater insight into their selves, which was more than enough to make them enthusiastic students.

This calls into question the traditional teaching method of just doing the form. Xu's real success as a motivator was his ability to relate stories from his students' own lives. As a youthful man in his 60s, when Xu explained how his students can become distracted by thoughts of their grandchildren that might cause them to miss a step and incur a fall, they saw the value of "being in the moment." Showing how T'ai Chi kept them in the moment occurred by his explanation, not merely by his demonstration of a move. While some may complain that that's spoon-feeding, it's also what kept more than the hard core in the class.

This study reveals the value of learning only part of the form—a benefit to many older people who have a hard time remembering moves, as the form grows longer and more complex. It's not condescending, but rather an explanation of why it's okay not to torture yourself over slow progress or frustration at learning new moves. When students are encouraged to see the value of what they already know, they're less frustrated by feelings of inadequacy. In fact, building self-esteem is a significant benefit to T'ai Chi study. The T'ai Chi students had a greatly improved sense of control over their own health. Given the growing body of evidence for the power of positive thinking, this is hardly surprising. Without trying to deny the impact of objective physical maladies, there's a lot of validity in the maxim: You're as healthy as you think you are. T'ai Chi gives people confidence that they can move in ways they might have been afraid to try without this training. By so doing, T'ai Chi builds the confidence that leads to more independent and thus more fulfilling lives.

The study's short length (only 10 weeks) also belies the fallacy that it takes years to benefit from T'ai Chi. While it's true that the T'ai Chi journey is a lifetime affair, it behooves teachers to emphasize that the benefits accrue from the first lesson. While serious T'ai Chi study cultivates humility, it's hardly appropriate in the early stages of study. The common statement that "I still know only very little" is a statement of philosophy, a recognition that there is still a long way to go on the T'ai Chi journey.

Studies such as this one present both an opportunity and a responsibility to everyone interested in Eastern thought and practice. We need to take advantage of good news such as this to show people that T'ai Chi works not just from our own Eastern flavored view of the world, but also when seen through the eyes of Western medical scientists.

While it's true, to paraphrase Lao Tzu, that "words can't reveal the whole truth," words can guide people in the right direction. T'ai Chi won't become the next fad, and will be healthier for that.

Medical Benefits of T'ai Chi: Articles

Following are some article summaries from both popular and professional journals and magazines that explore the medical effects of T'ai Chi practice. They cover the gamut of benefits from blood pressure and arthritis reduction to sports visualization and gestalt therapy.

General Benefits: "[T'ai Chi] teaches inner strength while toning muscles, increasing flexibility, and boosting immune power. It is also said to reduce stress, store up energy, increase body awareness, and improve balance and coordination. T'ai Chi was the closely held secret of a few Chinese families for nearly 1,000 years." (*Men's Health* magazine. 8 Mar/Apr 1993, 66–69.)

Physiological Benefits: "Relative to measurement beforehand, practice of T'ai Chi raised heart rate, increased nonadrenaline excretion in urine, and decreased salivary cortisol concentration. Relative to baseline levels, [test subjects] reported less tension, depression, anger, fatigue, confusion, and state-anxiety; they felt more vigorous, and in general they had less total mood disturbance." (American Psychological Association. *Journal of Psychosomatic Research.* 33 (2) (1989) 197–206.)

Mental Homeostasis: "Psychological homeostasis refers to emotional control or tranquility. It has been stated that the biological function of human emotion and repression is primarily homeostatic. Evidence suggests that a feedback relationship exists between forms of homeostasis, and the body-mind type of therapies (including acupuncture and T'ai Chi) thus have a combined physiological, physical, and psychological effect." (American Psychological Association. *American Journal of Chinese Medicine* 9 (1): 1–14 (Spring 1981).)

Immune System: "A study conducted in China indicates that T'ai Chi may increase the number of T lymphocytes in the body. Also know as T-Cells, these lymphocytes help the immune system destroy bacteria and possibly even tumor cells." (*Prevention Magazine.* Vol. 42, May 1990, p.14–15.)

Breathing, Aches, Blood Pressure: "Participants observed a 'big increase in breathing capacity,' a disappearance of backaches and neck aches, those with high blood pressure claimed a drop of 10 to 15 mm Hg systolic at rest, and all participants claimed to have more energy in their daily work." (*Hawaii Medical Journal.* 51 (8) (August 1992).)

Balance: "A 10-year study on aging through Harvard, Yale, and Emory University determined not only that T'ai Chi was superior to more technological balance therapies, but also that T'ai Chi reduced the risk of injury by falling by 48 percent. Complications from these injuries are the sixth leading cause of death in older Americans, and account for about $10 billion loss per year to the economy." (*USA Today.* May 1996.)

Mental and Physical Stress: "Mind and body exercises, such as...T'ai Chi...are increasingly replacing high-impact aerobics, long distance running, and other body punishing exercises of the 1980s...Mind/body workouts are kinder to the joints and muscles...reduce the tension that often contributes to the development of disease, which makes them especially appropriate for high powered, stressed out baby boomers. Unlike most conventional exercises, these forms are intended to stretch, tone, and relax the whole body instead of isolating parts...based on a series of progressive choreographed movements coordinated with deep breathing." (*Working Woman Magazine.* V 20 Feb. 1995, 60–62+.)

Postural Control: "T'ai Chi, a traditional Chinese exercise, is a series of individual dance-like movements linked together in a continuous, smooth-flowing sequence...An analysis of variance (ANOVA) demonstrated that in 3 of 5 tests, the T'ai Chi practitioners had significantly better postural control than the sedentary non practitioners." (*American Journal of Occupational Therapy.* 46 (4): 295–300 (April 1992).)

Beyond Traditional Care: "Health practitioners encountering clients who are faced with problems that do not seem to respond to traditional health care...may employ some of the health traditions of other cultures and to view the body and mind as a balanced whole. Massage, acupuncture and T'ai Chi...focus on the mind/body connection to facilitate healing through relaxation, pressure points, and movement." (*AAOHN Journal* 41 (7): 349–351 (July 1993).)

Cures/Preventions: "Proponents claim that T'ai Chi can also (1) cure illnesses such as hypertension, asthma, and insomnia; (2) prevent arteriosclerosis and spinal deformity, and (3) shorten recovery phase from long-term illness. Results from a study by Chen Munyi (1963) with elderly T'ai Chi practitioners show that this group had RTs, strength, and flexibility superior to nonpractitioners." (American Psychological Association. *American Journal of Chinese Medicine* 9 (1): 15–22 (Spring 1981).)

Balance: "Institute of Chicago indicates that people with moderate balance problems can be helped by practicing T'ai Chi. Participants...of the 2-month course...experienced about a 10 percent improvement in balance. An Emory University study supports Hain's findings." (*Prevention Magazine*. V. 46 December 1994, 71–72.)

Rheumatoid Arthritis: "No significant exacerbation of joint symptoms using this weight bearing system of exercises (T'ai Chi) was observed. T'ai Chi exercises appear to be safe for RA patients...weight bearing exercises have the potential advantages of stimulating bone growth and strengthening connective tissue. (*American Journal of Physical Medicine and Rehabilitation* 70 (3): 136–141 (June 1991).)

Support Groups Recommending T'ai Chi: Multiple Sclerosis, Fibromyalgia, Parkinson's Disease, Lupus, Migraines, Chronic Pain, AIDS: "Proper exercise [for AIDS sufferers] is typified by T'ai Chi. Dr. Laurence E. Badgley, M.D.

Psychology: "T'ai Chi is a natural and safe vehicle for both clients and staff to learn and experience the benefits of being able to channel, concentrate and co-ordinate their bodies and minds: to learn to relax and to 'neutralize' rather than resist the stress in their personal lives. This is an ability that we greatly need to nurture in our modern fast-paced society." (Dr. John Beaulieu, N.D., M.T.R.S. Bellevue Psychiatric Hospital, New York. [Refer to the book *The Supreme Ultimate* for full text].)

T'ai Chi and Gestalt Therapy: "Discussion of T'ai Chi, a Chinese system of integrated exercises, as an effective adjunct to Gestalt Therapy." (American Psychological Association. *Journal of Contemporary Psychotherapy* 10 (1): 25–31 (Fall 1978).)

Psychosomatic Illness: "A holistic paradigm, T'ai Chi, is proposed as a theoretical basis for treating psychosomatic illness." (American Psychological Association. *Journal of Black Psychology* 7 (1): 27–43 (August 1980).)

T'ai Chi Helps Understand Change: "Suggests the imagery of the T'ai Chi figure...can serve as a model for understanding the processes of change within psychotherapy. The T'ai Chi figure expresses the themes of unity and completeness, the dynamic of interplay and balance of opposite forces, and the cyclical nature of therapeutic change." (American Psychological Association. *Psychologia, An International Journal of Psychology in the Orient* 34 (1): 18–27 (MArch 1991).)

Elderly: "According to T'ai Chi enthusiasts, the discipline can prevent many ailments, including high blood pressure, tuberculosis, and diabetes, and U.S. scientists agree that T'ai Chi can offer some important fitness benefits, particularly for older adults." (*Modern Maturity.* V. 35 June/July 1992, 60–62.)

Cardiorespiratory Effects: "Conclusion: The data substantiate that practicing T'ai Chi regularly may delay the decline of cardiorespiratory function in older individuals. In addition, TC may be prescribed as a suitable aerobics exercise for older adults." (*Journal of American Geriatric Society* 43 (11): 1222–1227 (November 1995) ISSN: 0002-8614 Journal Code: H6V.)

Sports Health: "[Former] Boston Celtic's star Robert Parish, who, at age 39, is the oldest player in the NBA, credits the ancient martial art of T'ai Chi with his durability. Parish remains dominant in his 17th season in the league, and he has no plans to retire. He started all 79 games that he played last year for the Celtics, averaging 14.1 points, shooting 54 percent from the field and 77 percent from the free throw line, and racking up a season total of 705 rebounds and 97 blocked shots. (*Gentlemen's Quarterly.* V. 62 December 1992, 256–60.)

"Inspired by his success, fellow Celtics players Reggie Lewis and Rick Fox have signed on with Li (Parish's T'ai Chi instructor)." (*Gentlemen's Quarterly.* March 13, 1999.)

When Does T'ai Chi *Not* Work?

Although there are very few occasions when the practice of T'ai Chi can be considered dangerous, it is necessary to list those rare situations in order to protect the student from an unfortunate injury.

The primary consideration would be the health of the knee joints. Because the regular T'ai Chi and Qigong stances use a slightly bent knee, anyone with torn cartilage or other knee injuries should be extra careful not to overextend the knee.

Arthritis in the knee is not necessarily an expulsion from T'ai Chi practice. The secret is to go slowly, don't overextend your limits, and stop at the first sign of pain in the joint.

High blood pressure or cardiovascular weakness should not be a limiting factor, again as long as a degree of moderation is practiced.

Another point concerning T'ai Chi is related to its healing abilities. Just as Western medicine and surgery is not 100-percent effective in all cases, so too with T'ai Chi. For a small percentage of people, T'ai Chi will be either impossible to perform, even with adaptations, because of the severity of their afflictions, or it will have no observable healing effects. This could be due to improper practice techniques or not incorporating breathing into the movements. Regardless of the reasons, it is vitally important to remember that Western and Eastern modalities should be combined to create the perfect health regimen.

Chapter 11

Tao Now, Brown Cow

Taoism:
The Philosophy of T'ai Chi

A Definition of Taoist Philosophy

What exactly is Taoism, and why on earth is it important to know about it? You came here to learn T'ai Chi, not some crazy chanting religion, right?

Actually, that's wrong. The basis of T'ai Chi and Qigong, in addition to Traditional Chinese Medicine (TCM), is the Taoist philosophy. By gaining an understanding, however rudimentary, of the principles of Taoist thought, we can better appreciate *why* we do what we do when we practice our T'ai Chi. You could practice Wave Hands Like Clouds for your entire life without studying Taoism, true; but how much better it becomes when you know *why* the imagery of clouds is used in this exercise, why we use both hands at the same time, and why each exercise has a little psychological significance involved.

A basic working definition of Taoism, at least for our purposes, would be *the individual's search for balance, contentment, and health by attempting to "align" themselves with the universe*. This universe can be as big as the known universe, or it can be as small as your house or apartment. The alignment occurs through exercise, diet, meditation, medicine, and attitude adjustment. When you are balanced in thought as well as in body, you can be said to be in alignment with the Tao.

But what *is* the Tao?

A Philosophy or a Religion?

Translated loosely from Chinese, Tao means "way" or "path." So a Taoist is seeking and following a path through life. The particular path that an individual follows will vary from others' paths, but if successfully traveled, will result in becoming "in tune" with the world and everything and everyone within it. A noble goal, surely, but difficult! As the wise men say, "It's the journey, not the destination, that is important." So Taoists always consider how their actions will affect their journey, refusing to perform any task that draws them from their ultimate goal of self-mastery and integration into the world.

So if Tao is a path, what is Taoism? Is it simply following a path? Or is there more involved?

A little more. There are thousands of books and manuscripts in what is called the Taoist canon, the collected works of hundreds of authors over thousands of years. This body of work is considered essential study material for Taoist scholars, but we can take a condensed version along on our journey. The first consideration is whether Taoism is a religion or a philosophy. The answer? It's both, but it started as a philosophy. Only over time, with the influx of other belief systems and religions into China, did Taoism adopt religious trappings in order to compete with the new kids on the block.

When did Taoism start? Probably with the first caveman who saw lightning in the sky, or observed how water carried a fallen branch downstream. Og (to give him a name) began to draw conclusions from his observations: If he stayed in his cave, the bright light in the sky wouldn't hit him as it did that tree, nor would he fall into the river, nor would he end up far away from where he started. What Og was doing was forming the rudiments of a life philosophy—learning to go along with Nature in order to survive. This is the core teaching of Taoism—learn to blend with Nature, not fight it. Thus, Taoism could be said to have been one of the earliest Pagan or Nature-oriented beliefs in the world.

The religious form of Taoism is filled with gods and goddesses, warrior/scholar heroes, ceremonies for everything from the birth of a baby to the opening of a new store, days of festivals and celebrations, beautiful temples, prayer, meditation—in short, a religion in its own right. They have their own priests and nuns, who often reside in monasteries, as well as lay practitioners who attend to the everyday religious needs of the local population.

We'll examine more concepts of Taoism later in this chapter, but, for now, it is enough to know that our discussion of Taoism will be confined to the philosophical points and not the religious, so you don't need to worry about changing your faith. In fact, many of my students comment on how studying Taoist philosophy has helped them understand their own belief systems better and deeper. It allows them to become better people through introspection and meditation, and relieves much anxiety brought about through stressful lifestyles.

How Does Taoism Relate to T'ai Chi?

The Taoist philosophy is the guiding principle behind T'ai Chi—indeed, T'ai Chi was created by observing Nature in action. Remember the story about the snake and the crane fighting? The observation and subsequent reflection on that fight was what created T'ai Chi: an attempt to imitate the movements and strategies of animals.

Performed properly, T'ai Chi is a beautiful, nonstressful series of movements that flow into each other and seem never-ending. So, too, is Nature—she's beautiful (until we deviate from the Tao, or path, and pollute her); she is relaxing (spend a day walking in the woods or at the shore—relaxing, isn't it?); she ebbs and flows with the changing of the seasons and the constant cycle of day and night. So T'ai Chi in one sense can be said to be an attempt to mirror Nature by imitating her ways. I bet you never thought you were being a philosopher when you practiced Plate of Spaghetti!

So besides the constant change and motion of Nature being reflected in the smooth movements of T'ai Chi, what are some other parallels? Not to expend effort in doing things. Nature seems to accomplish her miracles with no effort: *poof*, a beautiful sunset; *voilà*, a flock of birds all turn at the same time. There is no force used in making these miracles occur, nor is there any great mental preparation or anxiety. It just happens spontaneously. So, too, should your T'ai Chi—the movements should reflect a certain ease of manner, gracefulness, and surety of action. When you practice your Cat Stepping, be as lithe and nimble as a cat. When you root yourself down in Marching in Place, be a mountain, strong and immovable. Flow like water whatever you are doing, and you will be one step closer to being in tune with your world.

Have you ever tried to do something that just didn't seem to want to get done? I have. What is your first reaction when you try and try and try, but it won't work? Frustrating, isn't it? It's like trying to pound a nail into an old, solid piece of oak. You bang and sweat and cuss, but the nail keeps bending or skipping away. You hit your thumb with the hammer and let loose with a stream of invectives. But the wood just sits there. You get a bigger hammer—no good. A bigger nail—still no good. The oak stands strong before your onslaught.

But what's this? A drill? With a tungsten carbide drill bit? Let's see…gee, that went into the wood like a hot knife into butter. Let's try that nail again—wow, that was easy!

What just happened? You tried and tried, but failed miserably. You took another course of action, and everything fell into place with hardly any effort. Did the wood change? Does Nature? Does your world? Yes, little things change, but their nature remains solid. This is an example of the soft overcoming the hard, as when water wears down a huge boulder in the stream over decades of rapid movement. You used a hard approach at first ("I'm going to drive this nail into the wood if it kills me!"). When that didn't work, you took a break and tried a soft way (using a drill is actually using mechanical advantage, another link with T'ai Chi's principles). Success! So the T'ai Chi principles Soft Overcomes Hard and Meet Advancement With Retreat illustrate the Taoist yin-yang principle of everything needing a complementary partner, and of learning to "go with the flow" in order to achieve success in life.

Basic Tenets of Taoism

Taoism, like any other belief system, has certain guiding principles that make it what it is. Here we will examine the basics, and as we do so, try to imagine how each principle relates to your T'ai Chi practice.

Tao Te Jing

The Chinese symbol for Tao is a combination of two separate symbols: one representing a human head, and one representing the act of walking. Thus, one interpretation is "walking a path of wisdom." This is the quintessential definition of Taoism: learning to walk the path or way.

"Te" is a Chinese word meaning "virtue." Its symbol combines three separate symbols representing "heart," "straight," and "to go." Thus, the title of the main work of Taoist thought, the Tao Te Jing, translates to "Walking the Path That Leads Straight from the Heart." This is an indication that a true Taoist will be himself and never deny his own nature. Rather, he will seek to become closer with the universal nature of everything and everybody.

Seeing Clearly

A Taoist will seek to see everything as it truly is, without embellishment or falsehoods. Piercing through the veil of illusions that we call life is but one of many activities that a follower of the Tao participates in.

Knowing Yourself

To understand *who* and *what* you are is a special quest of the Taoist. This speaks to the Seeing Clearly principle, in that you need to know yourself in order to function in the most natural fashion possible.

Detachment and Nonjudgmental

Taoists are not the type to judge others. It is not their place to do so, nor does it advance their own spiritual quest. They remain apart from material things, recognizing their needs and distinguishing them from their wants.

Not Trying But Doing

Taoists don't try; they do, or they don't. Kind of like Yoda from *Star Wars*. In fact, the creator of the Yoda character used Taoist thought for many of the wise old master's comments. "Trying" implies effort, strife, and the possibility of failure. A true Taoist will not accept these limitations.

Thinking Independently

Taoists are known for being independent thinkers, not followers of the crowd. I often use the term "Wolf or Sheep"—do you move and think with the common crowd, or do you stand apart?

Expanding the Self

Taoists seek to be open to all and to everything. They place no limits on compassion or love, but engage fully in understanding and spiritually recognizing all other beliefs. They are not held captive to a single way.

Faith In Life

It is all too easy to become pessimistic, the more we experience the bad parts of life. But what differentiates people of the Tao is that they don't lose faith in their lives. They do not fear change, understanding that it is a natural function of living, and welcome the opportunity to experience and learn new things every day.

Right Here, Right Now

Taoists are not paralyzed by a fear of the unknown of the future, nor are they caught looking backward longingly into the past. They realize that "right here, right now" is all we have to work with, so we should make it the best present moment that we can.

Enjoying Life

Taoists enjoy life to the utmost of their abilities. They know that our time here is short and that going through life mad and sad at everything is a waste of life. They joyously participate in the suffering, as well as the happiness of life.

Laughter

There's nothing wrong with laughing. In fact, it helps us deal with adversity and allows us a greater world view. In seeing the light side of things, we maintain an even perspective.

Nature

Taoists love nature. How could they do any less? They are part of it. In recognizing the wonders of nature, they learn about themselves. The greatest goal of a Taoist may very well be to become one with Nature, to feel the rhythms, ebbs, and flows of life in an intuitive fashion.

Nonresistance

Taoism advocates seeking the path of least resistance in life. Why butt your head against the wall when you can simply walk around it? This is intimately related to the act of nonstriving and being a natural person.

Using Taoism in Everyday Life

So how does all of this philosophy apply to you, dear reader? It applies quite strongly, even if you don't realize it yet. In practicing Taoism, you become a better person, both for yourself and for your loved ones. You shed the petty grievances and character flaws and learn to be more compassionate, loving, caring, and generally fun to be around.

How can you apply some of the Taoist principles to your everyday life?

For the past 2,000 years, traditional Western thinking has been dominated by a dualistic, either-or approach: either something is good, or it is bad; desirable or undesirable; someone is an ally or an enemy. We perceive experiences to be either positive or negative and we expend much energy in trying to eradicate that which we consider to be negative. From a Taoist point of view, this is like trying to erase the negative current from electricity because it is not positive.

Because we perceive ourselves as separate from others, we often find ourselves in opposition to them, locked into "this and that," merely because of skin color, language, or beliefs. Taking these "differences" for the way things "really are" leads to arguing, fighting, and even killing—all because of "this and that." We do the same with ourselves. We dislike parts of ourselves and struggle to change, not trusting that our own inner nature will of its own accord move towards a harmonious balance.

By being yielding and receptive, by remaining in relationship with others as well as with ourselves, we learn to flow with life's myriad changes. Indeed, we become an agent of change ourselves, rather than resisting it while desperately clinging to one experience or perception or the other.

"What goes up must come down," and "Every cloud has a silver lining." Our own language echoes the wisdom found within the concept of yin-yang. Bad luck becomes good luck and crisis contains the opportunity for growth. We can choose to cooperate with this complement of opposites by not denying, suppressing, or struggling against unwanted discomfort or pain, but rather by accepting all facets of our existence, good and bad, as the natural flow of the Tao.

By following the path of acceptance and responsiveness to change we can become, in the words of the Taoist philosopher Chuang Tzu, "true women and men of Tao." The true person of Tao "is not always looking for right and wrong, always deciding 'Yes' or 'No.' The true person has no mind to fight Tao and does not try by her own contriving to help Tao along. All that comes out of him comes quiet, like the four seasons."

The essential message of Taoism is that life constitutes an organic, interconnected whole that undergoes constant transformation. This unceasing flow of change manifests itself as a natural order governed by unalterable, yet perceivable laws. Strangely enough, it is the constancy of these governing principles (like the rising and setting of the sun and moon and the changing of the seasons) that allows people to recognize and utilize them in their own process of transformation. Gaining an awareness of life's essential unity and learning to cooperate with its natural flow and order enables people to attain a state of being that is both fully free and independent and at the same time fully connected to the life flow of the universe— being at one with the Tao. From the Taoist viewpoint this represents the ultimate stage of human existence.

The writings of the legendary Taoist sages Lao Tzu and Chuang Tzu furnish us with specific principles as a guide to attaining this state of oneness. Through understanding these principles and applying them to daily living, we may unconsciously become a part of life's flow.

A key principle in realizing our oneness with the Tao is that of wu-wei, or nondoing. Wu-wei refers to behavior that arises from a sense of oneself as connected to others and to one's environment. It is not motivated by a sense of separateness. It is action that is spontaneous and effortless. At the same time, it is not to be considered inertia, laziness, or mere passivity. Rather, it is the experience of going with the grain or swimming with the current. Our contemporary expression "going with the flow" is a direct expression of this fundamental Taoist principle, which, in its most basic form, refers to behavior occurring in response to the flow of the Tao.

The principle of wu-wei contains certain implications. Among these is the need to consciously experience ourselves as part of the unity of life that is the Tao. Lao Tzu writes that we must be quiet and watchful, learning to listen to both our own inner voices and to the voices of our environment in a noninterfering, receptive manner. In this way we also learn to rely on more than just our intellect and logical mind to gather and assess information. We develop and trust our intuition as our direct connection to the Tao. We heed the intelligence of our whole body, not only our brain. And we learn through our own experience. All of this allows us to respond readily to the needs of the environment, which of course includes ourselves. And just as the Tao functions in this manner to promote harmony and balance, our own actions, performed in the spirit of wu-wei, produce the same result.

Wu-wei also implies action that is spontaneous, natural, and effortless. As with the Tao, this behavior simply flows through us because it is the right action, appropriate to its time and place, and serving the purpose of greater harmony and balance. Chuang Tzu refers to this type of being in the world as flowing, or more poetically as "purposeless wandering!" How opposite this concept is to some of our most cherished cultural values. To have no purpose is unthinkable and even frightening, certainly anti-social, and perhaps pathological in the context of modern-day living. And yet it would be difficult to maintain that our current values have promoted harmony and balance, either environmentally or on an individual or social level.

To allow yourself to "wander without purpose" can be frightening because it challenges some of our most basic assumptions about life, about who we are as humans, and about our roles in the world. From a Taoist point of view, it is our cherished beliefs—that we exist as separate beings, that we can exercise willful control over all situations, and that our role is to conquer our environment—that lead to a state of disharmony and imbalance. Yet, "the Tao nourishes everything," Lao Tzu writes. If we can learn to follow the Tao, practicing "nonaction," then nothing remains undone. We should learn to trust our own bodies, our thoughts and emotions, and also believe that the environment will provide support and guidance. Thus, the need to develop watchfulness and quietness of mind.

In cultivating wu-wei, timing becomes an important aspect of our behavior. We learn to perceive processes in their earliest stage and thus are able to take timely action. "Deal with the small before it becomes large," is a well-known quote from Lao Tzu.

And finally, in the words of Chuang Tzu, we learn "detachment, forgetfulness of results, and abandonment of all hope of profit." By allowing the Tao to work through us, we make our actions truly spontaneous, natural, and effortless. We thus flow with all experiences and feelings as they come and go. We know intuitively that actions that are not ego-motivated, but are in response to the needs of the environment, lead harmonious balance and give ultimate meaning and purpose to our lives. Such actions are attuned to the deepest flow of life itself.

To allow wu-wei to manifest in our lives may seem like a difficult task. And yet, if we reflect on our past experiences, we will recall possibly many instances when our actions were spontaneous and natural, when they arose out of the needs of the moment without thought of profit or tangible result. "The work is done and then forgotten. And so it lasts forever," writes Lao Tzu.

By listening carefully within, as well as to our surroundings, by remembering that we are part of an interconnected whole, by remaining still until action is called forth, we can perform valuable, necessary, and long-lasting service in the world while cultivating our ability to be at one with the Tao. Such is the power of wu-wei, allowing ourselves to be guided by the Tao.

In the earliest Taoist written works, which appeared around 500 B.C., there are numerous references to the sage. From a Taoist viewpoint, this term refers to one whose actions are in complete harmony with his surroundings—both the immediate environment and the universe as a whole. Through the example of the sage, Taoism offers us a model of a way of being that is in accordance with the natural laws that govern life. To think and act like a sage is to attune oneself to life's flow and to the Tao.

In the English language, the word "sage" describes a wise person, one of sound judgment. It also means "to perceive keenly." Within the Taoist tradition, the sage has gained a wisdom that extends beyond mere intellectual knowledge or information and reflects a deep, intuitive understanding of life.

The sage expresses his wisdom by directly manifesting these principles in daily living. Because he truly experiences the unity of all life, the sage perceives and understands all opposites as part of the same system. As the sage does not oppose these opposites, they can bring harmony and balance to all situations. Because the sage resides in a state of interconnectedness, his actions do not arise from the needs of a separate age but are called forth by the needs of the environment, which includes the sage himself. These actions are natural, effortless, and spontaneous and are imbued with the power of the Tao.

Taoist thought maintains that cultivating sage-like attributes is part of the process of human transformation. While we may think that to become sage-like happens only at the final stage of this transformation, we also can recognize and foster those attributes already within us. The early Taoist writers, Lao Tzu and Chuang Tzu, themselves legendary sages, offer us numerous examples of behavior based on sage-like virtues. Most well known are Lao Tzu's "three treasures": compassion, frugality, and humility.

"Whoever has compassion can be brave. Whoever has frugality can be generous. Whoever dares not to be first in the world can become leader of the world." Lao Tzu maintains that these values are foreign neither to our understanding, nor to our experience, and that we are all capable of cultivating such sage-like characteristics because they are a natural part of being human. It is through our caring that we connect with others and with all of life. By practicing frugality, we maintain a balanced existence with our environment and develop simplicity in action and thought. And by learning to follow, we determine the needs of the environment and provide the necessary service.

The sage, in "perceiving keenly," sees past the dualities of right and wrong, and harmonizes all opposites. Lao Tzu states, "The sage is good to people who are good. He is also good to people who are not good." This is true goodness. The sage does not judge, but accepts everything as part of the intrinsic flow of life, and then acts accordingly. In this manner he (or she) provides the opportunity for all beings to become aware of their own self-worth and to express this as goodness.

The sage lives her life not by conventional standards, but according to the principles that are a reflection of the Tao. Chuang Tzu writes, "Rank and reward make no appeal to her. Disgrace and shame do not deter her. She is not always looking for right and wrong." Thus the sage is truly at peace with herself and with the way of the Tao. She believes that "the world is ruled by letting things take their course."

Chuang Tzu also writes that, as we become attuned to the Tao by living in harmony with the natural order of the universe, we become fully realized beings, or "true persons."

"They took life as it came, gladly. Took death as it came, without care. They had no mind to fight Tao. They did not try, by their own contriving, to help Tao along. These are the ones we call true persons."

Thus, to live in harmony with the Tao, cooperating with the natural laws that govern the universe means to grow and transform as individuals, to become sage-like in our behavior. Initially this process occurs because we consciously adopt and follow those principles that reflect the workings of the Tao—yin-yang and wu-wei, among others. In time we find that our sage-like behaviors occur reflexively and naturally. They emerge from us without conscious effort. We reach what Taoism considers to be a person's highest calling—a life in service of the Tao. "The Sage has no mind of her own. She is simply aware of the needs of others." Just as the Tao "nourishes all things," as it continually returns things to harmony and balance, so too does the sage. And this is the ultimate expression of the natural wisdom, the "sageliness," that is the essence of our being.

Chapter 12

Take Two Lizards and Call Me in the Morning

Traditional Chinese Medicine and T'ai Chi

A Definition of Traditional Chinese Medicine

Traditional Chinese Medicine (TCM), or Oriental Medicine as it is sometimes called, evolved in China over a 5000-year period of consistent use, making it the oldest system of medicine still in use today. It also forms the traditional medicine of countries such as Korea and Japan and is widely practiced throughout the Western world in America, the United Kingdom, and parts of Europe and Australia.

TCM incorporates acupuncture, herbal medicine, massage, dietary therapy, and exercise systems such as T'ai Chi and Qigong to prevent and treat a wide range of acute and chronic conditions. We've already explored T'ai Chi and Qigong in the earlier chapters of this book, and in the third section of this chapter we'll explore each of the segments of TCM in more detail.

The underlying principle of TCM is that all living plants and animals contain a life force or energy that circulates continuously through them until they die. In humans, our life force (called Qi) circulates throughout channels or meridians, the main ones connecting with our internal organs. Basically, "perfect" health may be regarded as the smooth and unobstructed flow of Qi (and blood) throughout the body. When Qi and blood flow are obstructed, ill health results. Many factors contribute to this; hereditary, dietary, and environmental and lifestyle factors such as overworking and stress may all impede the flow of Qi and blood.

One of the major differences between TCM and Western medicine is that the former views the body from a holistic viewpoint. Mind, body, and spirit are inseparable, interconnecting with and influencing one another. Western medicine in comparison looks at the body from a scientific, microscopic point of view, isolating and treating each part as a separate entity with little recognition of its relationship to the whole.

TCM regards each of us as completely unique individuals. The TCM doctor looks for "patterns of disharmony," which are groups of symptoms and signs that are uniquely yours. Treatment is specifically tailored to suit your particular condition at that time. In contrast, the Western medicine doctor gives every patient with the same condition the same treatment without recognition of the fact that each patient is totally different from the next in virtually every regard.

Treatment for any complaint whether by acupuncture, herbs, or massage aims to restore inner harmony to the body by balancing energy and blood flow. When you visit a TCM doctor, he or she will ask you questions not only about your main complaint but also about other seemingly unrelated aspects of your health and lifestyle. What you eat, your sleeping patterns, bowel movements, type of work, emotions, menstrual irregularities, and many other details are noted during the initial consultation. Inspection of your tongue and palpation of the radial pulse on each of your wrists also provides important information with which to make a diagnosis.

Your initial visit can last up to an hour and may include acupuncture or massage therapy depending on your complaint. You may be prescribed a relevant herbal formula and be advised on appropriate dietary and lifestyle changes. We'll explore what is involved in TCM diagnosis in more detail later in this chapter.

TCM is increasingly being used by people in Western countries looking for alternatives to invasive and, in some cases, unnecessary surgical procedures, as well as for alternatives to modern pharmaceuticals that often produce unwanted side effects.

It may appear that I'm advocating TCM as the "one and only" healthcare system. Not so. Both TCM and Western medicine have advantages and limitations, and, in fact, the best results are often obtained from combining the two. For example, in Chinese hospitals, cancer patients are treated with chemotherapy and radiation but they are also given herbal medicine to combat the debilitating side effects of their treatment. This means that higher doses of chemotherapy and radiation can be tolerated by the patient, making the overall treatment more effective. To use another example: If I broke my leg, obviously the first place I would want to go to is a hospital. But I would make use of TCM modalities such as acupuncture to reduce the pain and speed up the healing process.

TCM works by stimulating the self-healing powers of the body and eliminating the root cause of a disease or ailment. Natural methods take time though, and while they lack the dramatic impact of modern medicines, they work in harmony with the body; therefore, the benefits are long lasting and side effects are rare.

In Western countries, acupuncture is probably the most widely recognized of the TCM modalities. The following is a list of conditions generally thought to respond best to acupuncture treatment:

∞ Acute strains and sprains of muscles and joints.

∞ Chronic neck and back pain.

∞ Headache.

∞ Constipation.

∞ Diarrhea.

∞ Indigestion.

∞ High blood pressure.

∞ Menstrual irregularities.

∞ Impotence.

∞ Post-stroke paralysis.

∞ Addictions such as overeating, smoking, and drug dependence.

This is by no means a definitive list.

An increasing number of experts from different areas of healthcare believe that the most effective medicines of the future will combine the "best of both worlds." By utilizing modern Western procedures and traditional therapies such as acupuncture and Chinese herbal medicine, more effective results can be achieved.

Privately run multi-modality clinics of this nature have been operating in countries such as America and Australia for some time, but until we see signs such as "TCM Department" in the corridors of our major hospitals will we know that true acceptance of natural therapies in the West has arrived.

How Does TCM relate to T'ai Chi?

All of the principles of Taoism that we examined in the last chapter, as well as some that we did not, apply to both TCM and T'ai Chi. Based on the yin-yang principle, TCM seeks to balance the body. Take, for example, a fever. Often, the methods of TCM will induce yet a higher fever, albeit temporarily, in order to lead it into a balanced state. This is explained by the principle of "lead an unbalanced condition into yet a more unbalanced state, and it will seek to gain equilibrium." In other words, start with a fever, make it even more feverish, and it will, by its own nature, want to return to a normal, healthy state. T'ai Chi seeks to portray and practice the same principle. When you are performing Set the Waves Rolling in the 18-Movement Qigong Form, you are trying to determine how far forward you can push before you lose your balance. In experimenting with this movement, you ultimately discover that you need to keep your body upright and your weight rooted into the ground, and allow your hands to push only as far forward as is comfortable, usually not beyond your front toes. If you push too far, your body bends forward and downward, and you lose your balance. You have just learned about equilibrium, and how going too far in one direction will lead to a movement in the opposite one.

Another way to illustrate the bond between TCM and T'ai Chi is to look at the five Elements of Chinese medicine. Water, Earth, Wood, Fire, and Metal make up what is seen as the five primary Elements of all material in the universe. In TCM, an entire school of diagnosis and treatment is devoted to the Five Element style, wherein a balance of the five Elements is sought to alleviate sickness. Too much Water? Add some Fire. Too Woody? Add Metal. There is a complete cycle of creating and extinguishing among the five Elements, and to treat your patient using this principle, you need to know and use that cycle. The actual theory is beyond the scope of this book; it's only important that you get an idea of what is involved.

With T'ai Chi, the five Elements get to show their stuff! When you are showing Earth, you are rooted down, heavy, with a stable base; just like Mother Earth. Certainly, you show Water throughout the movements by your fluid style and lack of resistance. You are precise in your movements, like Metal, and stand upright and tall, like Wood. Fire? Perhaps that's your spirit when you do the T'ai Chi form with a martial attitude. Or perhaps it's the Qi rising and flowing throughout your body.

As we saw in the Qigong exercises, each movement has a relationship to an organ, an organ system, or to general Qi flow in the body. When you perform Qigong or T'ai Chi, you are practicing Chinese medicine! You are moving your body in a way that influences your health through the meridians and channels, as well as your physical health through the gentle flexing and bending of the joints.

Basic Components of TCM

Having already explored T'ai Chi and Qigong in earlier chapters, we will now look at the four other constituents of TCM—acupuncture, massage, herbs, and medical Qigong therapy.

Acupuncture

There are two very different ways of looking at acupuncture: from the traditional Chinese perspective and from the modern international perspective. Each of these will be briefly described.

Traditional View

The understanding of how acupuncture works has evolved with its practice, but the descriptions set down a thousand years ago have largely been retained. The dominant function of acupuncture is to regulate the circulation of Qi (vital energy) and blood.

Approximately 2,000 years ago, the preeminent acupuncture text, *Huangdi Neijing (Yellow Emperor's Classic on Internal Medicine)* was written. In it, acupuncture was described as a means of letting out excess Qi or blood by making holes in the body along certain pathways, called Jingluo (meridians). For some of these meridians, it was advised to acupuncture in such a way as to let out the blood but not the Qi; for others, to let out the Qi, but not the blood. Many diseases were thought to enter the body through the skin, and then penetrate inward through muscle, internal organs, and, if not cured in a timely fashion, to the bone marrow. By inserting a needle to the appropriate depth—to correspond with the degree of disease penetration—the disease could be let out.

Prior to the time when there were microscopes by which people could envision individual cells, and before autopsies revealed the intricate structures within the body, doctors and scholars projected the internal workings of the body from what they could actually experience, which was the world outside the body. On this basis, the workings of the body were described in terms similar to those used to describe the visible world. One of the critical aspects of nature for humans living a thousand years ago, when Chinese civilization was well developed, was the system of watercourses, which included tiny streams, huge rivers, manmade canals, and the ocean. It was envisioned that the body had a similar system of moving, life-giving fluid. This fluid was Qi, and the pathways through which it flowed were meridians.

Instead of discussing acupuncture in terms of letting something out of the body, physicians working a thousand years later described it in terms of regulating something within the body. The flow of Qi through the meridians, just like the flow of water through a stream, could be blocked off by an obstruction—a dam across the waterway. In the streams, this might be a fallen tree or a mudslide; in humans, it might be caused by something striking the body, the influence of bad weather, or ingestion of improper foods. When a stream is blocked, it floods above the blockage, and below the blockage it dries up. If one goes to the point of blockage and clears it away, then the stream can resume its natural course. In a similar manner, if the Qi in the meridian becomes blocked, the condition of the body becomes disordered like the dryness and flooding; if one could remove the blockage from the flow of Qi within a meridian, the natural flow could be restored.

In a blocked stream, just cutting a small hole or crevice in the blockage will often clear the entire stream path, because the force of the water that penetrates the hole will widen it continuously until the normal course is restored. In the human body, inserting a small needle into the blocked meridian will have a similar effect. Just as a stream may have certain points more easily accessed (or more easily blocked), the meridians have certain points that, if treated by needling, will have a significant impact on the flow pattern. Many acupuncture points are named for geological structures: mountains, streams, ponds, and oceans.

Although this description of the basic acupuncture concept is somewhat simplified, it conveys the approach that is taught today to students of traditional acupuncture: locate the areas of disturbance, isolate the main blockage points, and clear the blockage. Of course, many layers of sophistication have been added to this model, so that the needling—which might be carried out in several different ways—can be seen to have subtle and differing effects depending upon the site(s) needled, the depth and direction of needling, and even the chemical composition of the needle (such as gold, silver, or steel). For example, some needling techniques are used for the primary purpose of increasing the flow of Qi in a meridian without necessarily removing any blockage; other techniques reduce the flow of Qi in the meridians. These tonifying and draining methods, as well as transference methods that help move Qi from one meridian to another, are part of the more general aim of balancing the flow of Qi in the body.

Ultimately, all the descriptions of acupuncture that are based on the traditional model involve rectifying a disturbance in the flow of Qi. If the Qi circulation is corrected, the body can eliminate most symptoms and eventually—with proper diet, exercise, and other habits—overcome virtually all disease.

Modern Views

When the human body was finally described in terms of cells, biochemicals, and specific structures (most of this accomplished less than 150 years ago), the Chinese method of acupuncture and its underlying concepts were evaluated in these new terms. As a first effort, researchers sought out physical pathways that might correspond to the meridians, and even a fluid substance that might correspond to Qi. Neither of these was found. Nonetheless, the action of performing acupuncture was shown to have effects on the body that required some detailed explanation.

From the modern perspective, rather than blockages of circulation described in the old Chinese dogma, diseases are understood to be caused by microorganisms, metabolic failures, changes in DNA structure or signaling, or breakdown of the immune system. Some of these disorders are resolved by the cellular functions that are designed for healing, while others become chronic diseases because the pathological factors involved have either defeated the body's curing mechanisms or because something else has weakened the body's responses to the point that they are ineffective. For example, poor nutrition, unhealthy habits, and high stress can weaken the responses to disease.

Modern studies have revealed that acupuncture stimulates one or more of the signaling systems, which can, under certain circumstances, increase the rate of healing response. This may be sufficient to cure a disease, or it might only reduce its impact (alleviate some symptoms). These findings can explain most of the clinical effects of acupuncture therapy.

According to current understanding, the primary signaling system affected by acupuncture is the nervous system, which not only transmits signals along the nerves that comprise it, but also emits a variety of biochemicals that influence other cells of the body. The nervous system is connected to the hormonal system via the adrenal gland, and it makes connections to every cell and system of the body.

According to traditional Chinese doctors, one of the key elements of a successful acupuncture treatment is having the person who is being treated experience what is called the "needling sensation." This sensation may vary with the treatment, but it has been described as numbness, tingling, warmth, or other experience that is not simple pain (pain is not an expected or desired response to acupuncture treatment, though it is recognized that needling certain points may involve a painful response). Sometimes the needling sensation is experienced as propagating from the point of needling to another part of the body. The acupuncturist, while handling the needle, should experience a response called "getting Qi." In this case, the needle seems to get pulled by the body, and this may be understood in modern terms as the result of muscle responses secondary to the local nervous system interaction.

According to this interpretation, acupuncture is seen as a stimulus directed to certain responsive parts of the nervous system that set off a biochemical cascade that enhances healing. Some acupuncture points are very frequently used and their applications are quite varied: needling at these points may stimulate a "global" healing response that can affect many diseases. Other points have only limited applications; needling at those points may affect only one of the signaling systems. It is common for acupuncturists to combine the broad-spectrum points and the specific points for each treatment. Some acupuncturists come to rely on a few of these broad-spectrum points as treatments for virtually all common ailments.

This modern explanation of how acupuncture works does not explain why the acupuncture points are arrayed along the traditional meridian lines. At this time, no one has identified—from the modern viewpoint—a clear series of neural connections that would correspond to the meridians. However, acupuncturists have identified other sets of points, such as those in the outer ear, which seem to be mapped to the whole body.

The description, in the case of the ear, is of a layout of the body in the form of a "homunculus" (a miniature humanoid form). Such patterns might be understood more easily than the meridian lines, because the brain, which is adjacent to the ear, also has a homunculus pattern that has been identified by modern research.

Similarly, acupuncturists have identified zones of treatment (for example, on the scalp or on the hand) that correspond to large areas of the body, and this may also be more easily explained because there are connections from the spinal column to various parts of the body that might have secondary branches elsewhere. In fact, acupuncture by zones, homunculus, "ashi" points (places on the body that are tender and indicate a blockage of Qi circulation), and "trigger" points (spots that are associated with muscle groups) is becoming a dominant theme, as the emphasis on treating meridians fades. The new focus is on finding effective points for various disorders and for getting biochemical responses (rather than regulating Qi, though there is no doubt there is some overlap between the two concepts).

During this modern period (since the 1970s), an increasing number of ways to stimulate the healing response at various body points have been advocated, confirming that needling is not a unique method (the idea that the needle would produce a hole through which pathogenic forces could escape has long been fading). In the past, the main procedures for affecting acupuncture points were needling and application of heat (moxabustion).

Now there is increasing reliance on electrical stimulation (with or without needling) and laser stimulation. Because the basic idea of acupuncture therapy is gaining popularity throughout the world while the practice of needling is restricted to certain health professions and is not always convenient, other methods are also becoming widely used. Laypersons and practitioners with limited training are applying finger pressure (acupressure), tiny metal balls held to the skin by tape, magnets (with or without tiny needles attached), piezoelectric stimulus (a brief electric discharge), and low-energy electrical pulsing (such as the TENS unit provides with electrical stimulus applied to the skin surface by taped electrodes). Some of these methods may have limited effectiveness, but it appears that if an appropriate body site is stimulated properly, then the healing response is generated.

For many nervous system functions, timing is very important, and this is the case for acupuncture. The duration of therapy usually needs to be kept within certain limits (too short and no effect, too long and the person may feel exhausted), and the stimulation of the point is often carried out with a repetitive activity (maintained for a minute or two by manual stimulation—usually slight thrusting, slight withdrawing, or twirling—or throughout treatment with electrostimulation). It has been shown in laboratory experiments that certain frequencies of stimulus work better than others, as might be expected for nervous system responses, but not expected for simple chemical release from other cells.

Traditional and Modern Views Coexisting

The traditional and modern understandings of acupuncture arise from significantly different world views and from application of different levels of technology. It is difficult to directly correlate the two, though one can say that many of the traditional observations and ideas have partial explanations by modern mechanisms. Still, the modern practitioner can become aware of and trained in the application of both approaches to acupuncture. A person to be treated can be analyzed from both perspectives and the treatment strategy can be devised according to the conclusions derived from each perspective. Certain aspects of the case may be more amenable to traditional analysis and corresponding treatment, while other aspects are better suited to modern analysis and treatment approach.

An individual who is suffering from a chronic pain syndrome might be analyzed in terms of which meridians are blocked: through treatment of appropriate points on the meridian, the pain might be alleviated. The same individual might be analyzed according to which muscle groups are involved in the painful area and might be treated by acupuncture at points that specifically affect those muscles. An individual suffering from an autoimmune disorder might be analyzed according to which of the traditional organ systems are involved, with treatment of the associated meridians. The same individual might be analyzed in terms of the immune system disturbance and treated by stimulating points that have been identified as immune regulators.

Because the traditional acupuncture approach has been shown to be effective in clinical trials conducted in China (and elsewhere in Asia), one can rely on the traditional methods. However, many practitioners in the West, with little or no prior exposure to Oriental philosophy but with experience and training in Western modes of analysis, may feel uncomfortable turning partly or completely to the traditional Chinese view, and will, instead, focus on the modern understanding of this healing technique.

Herbs

(I'd like to thank Dr. Subhuti Dharmananda from the Institute for Traditional Medicine for his permission to use the following introduction to Chinese herbs.)

Chinese herbs, of which there are hundreds, are an ancient modality of healing. The herbal tradition of China is valued scientifically, as well as being a fascinating and popular tradition. Scientists working in China and Japan during the past four decades have demonstrated that the herb materials contain active components that can explain many of their claimed actions. Modern drugs have been developed from the herbs, such as treatments for asthma and hay fever from Chinese ephedra; hepatitis remedies from schizandra fruits and licorice roots; and a number of anticancer agents from trees and shrubs. Several popular formulations produced in China, called "patent medicines," are relied upon daily by millions of Chinese (in China and abroad), such as the Bupleurum Sedative Pills and Women's Precious Pills that invigorate the energy, nourish the blood, calm tension, and regulate menstruation, and Yin Chiao Jie Du Pian, which is a reliable treatment for the early stages of common cold, sore throat, and influenza.

More than 300 herbs that are commonly used today have a history of use that goes back at least 2,000 years. Over that time, a vast amount of experience has been gained that has gone toward perfecting their clinical applications. According to Chinese clinical studies, these herbs, and others that have been added to the list of useful items over the centuries, can greatly increase the effectiveness of modern drug treatments, reduce their side effects, and sometimes replace them completely.

In China, the two most common methods of applying herb therapies are to make a decoction (a strong tea that must be simmered for an hour or more) and to make large honey-bound pills (boluses). Both of these forms meet with considerable resistance in Western countries. The teas are deemed too time-consuming, smelly, and awful-tasting to justify their use, and the honey pills are sticky, difficult to chew, and bad tasting. Thus, modern forms that are more acceptable have been developed for most applications.

The two popular forms to replace the standard Chinese preparations are extract powders (or granules) and smooth, easy-to-swallow tablets or capsules. The extracts are made by producing a large batch of tea and then removing the water and producing a powder or tiny pellets; the resulting material is swallowed down with some water or mixed with hot water to make a tea. Tablets and capsules contain either powdered herbs or dried extracts or a combination of the two. Despite the convenience, one must take a substantial quantity of these prepared forms (compared to the amount of drugs one takes).

For example, doses of the dried extracts range from 1 to 2 teaspoons each time, two to three times per day, and the tablets or capsules range from about three to eight units each time, two to three times per day.

The herb materials used in all these preparations are gathered from wild supplies or cultivated, usually in China (some come from India, the Mid-East, or elsewhere). There are an estimated 6,000 species in use, including nearly 1,000 materials derived from animal sources and over 100 minerals, all of them categorized under the general heading "herbs." Herbs are processed in various ways, such as cleaning, soaking, slicing, and drying, according to the methods that have been reported to be most useful. These materials are then combined in a formulation; the ingredients and amounts of each item depend on the nature of the condition to be treated.

In some cases, a practitioner of Chinese medicine will design a specific formulation for an individual patient, which might be changed frequently over a course of treatment. In other cases, one or more formulas already prepared for ingestion without modification are selected for use. The outcome is monitored, and the determination of whether to continue the current formula, change to another, or discontinue use is made on the basis of actual versus desired outcomes and the obvious or subtle effects of using the herbs.

As a general rule, acute ailments (those that arise suddenly and are to be treated right away) are treated for a period of one to 30 days. If an outbreak of influenza or eruption of herpes virus is caught early enough, a one- or two-day treatment will prevent further development of the disease. In the case of acute active hepatitis causing jaundice, a treatment of 15 to 30 days may be necessary. For chronic diseases (those that have persisted for several months or years), the treatment time is often dependent on the dosage used and the ability of the individual to undertake all necessary steps to overcome the disease (perhaps changing diet, lowering stress, and increasing exercise). When a high-dosage therapy is applied, most chronic ailments can come under control (and some are cured) by a treatment of about three months' duration. If the daily dosage is lowered (because of inability to take the higher doses), the treatment time increases—perhaps to six to 12 months. Examples of chronic ailments are autoimmune disorders and degenerative diseases associated with aging. In some cases, herbs are taken daily, for an indefinite period, just as some drugs are taken daily. This is typically the situation when there are genetic disorders or permanent damage that cannot be entirely reversed, problems of aging, and ailments that have been left for too long without effective treatment.

The main reason that more Westerners are turning to Chinese herbs rather than local herbs is because of the vast scope of experience in using the Chinese materials. In every province of China, there are large schools of traditional Chinese medicine, research institutes, and teaching hospitals, where thousands of practitioners each year gain training in the use of herbs. The written heritage of Chinese medicine is quite rich. Ancient books are retained, with increasing numbers of commentaries. New books are written by practitioners who have had several decades of personal experience or by compilers who scan the vast diverse modern literature and arrange the results of clinical trials into neat categories.

American practitioners are usually trained at any one of about 45 colleges in the United States, with a three- or four-year series of courses that include basic Oriental medical theory, acupuncture, and herb prescribing. Certification is offered at the national level and licensing or registration is offered now by most states. Many doctors from China have come to the United States and currently offer professional services throughout the country, but most often in the larger cities. Continuing education is provided through numerous symposia offered by the colleges and professional organizations devoted to Oriental medicine. Often, these meetings focus on the treatment of specific diseases or training in the use of a specialized acupuncture technique or valuable herb formula.

Chinese herbs are provided in the United States as food supplements, not as drugs. Thus, they are not strictly regulated by the FDA except for monitoring the cleanliness of manufacturing facilities (for those materials made in the U.S.; for imported items, the FDA monitors only the listing of ingredients to help ensure no toxic herbs are being used). Random testing of crude herb materials and herb products made in the United States indicate that they are free of harmful bacteria and chemical contaminants. Imported products must be used with some caution, as some of them are problematic, yet get past the investigators. There are a few patent remedies that are labeled with only herb ingredients, but also contain several Western drugs. Some patents from China contain only Western drugs (and say so on the box, in Chinese), but purchasers may be unaware of this because they are told only that this is an effective remedy that came from China. Thus, imported Chinese herb products should be taken solely on the basis of a prescription from a trained health professional.

Negative interactions with Western drugs have not been noted for any of the common herb materials when used in the normal dosage range. A few people experience allergic reaction to individual herbs, a problem that often cannot be predicted in advance because these are idiosyncratic responses. A more common reaction is a gastrointestinal response, which might include constipation or diarrhea, nausea or bloating. Such reactions may occur if the individual has poor digestive functions, or if the herbal formula is not quite right for the needs of the individual. Taking the herbs at a different time in relation to meals may be helpful in resolving some of the gastrointestinal reactions. In a few cases, use of Chinese herb formulas may cause dizziness, headache, agitation, sleepiness, hunger, decreased appetite, sensation of heat or cold, or other sensory reactions. If such responses persist after about three days of using the herbs, it may be necessary to change formulas.

Most American practitioners find themselves too busy (because of the small number of practitioners in this country) to prepare detailed reports of their successful cases; thus, it is necessary to rely primarily on the large-scale clinical trials conducted in China to learn about the success rates. Such clinical reports, published in the Chinese language, are abstracted and published in English by the Chinese University of Hong Kong.

Massage

Chinese massage, or Tui Na as it is called, is a healing modality older than even acupuncture and herbs. It all began when prehistoric man discovered an ache on his body, began to (instinctively) rub it, and found that it felt better as a result. This ancient Chinese bodywork is now gaining rapid acceptance in the Western world.

Tui Na (pronounced twee-nah) massage is a complete healing system, like acupuncture and Chinese herbal medicine. It is probably the oldest system of bodywork still practiced, yet its popularity continues to grow.

Massage as a part of Chinese medical treatment goes back about 4,000 years. Written massage textbooks began to appear as early as the 4th century B.C., along with the earliest Chinese medical texts. Massage appears to have developed alongside both therapeutic exercise (Qigong) and acupuncture, as it depends on the same understanding of the meridians and the flow of Qi in the human body. The type of massage known as Qi healing, or curing with external Qi (Medical Qigong Therapy), was developed by Master teachers of Qigong.

Benefits

Chinese massage is not intended to be an experience of pampering or relaxation. It is a form of deep tissue therapy that conveys the following benefits:

- Speeding the healing of injuries and clearing bruises.
- Stimulating blood circulation and regulating the nervous system.
- Removing scar tissue.
- Easing emotional distress.
- Curing some conditions affecting the internal organs.

so Increasing flexibility in the joints and improving posture.

so Relieving chronic pain.

so Maintaining wellness and functioning as a form of preventive care.

so Improving athletic performance.

so Strengthening the body's resistance to disease.

Some forms of Chinese massage do not require extensive training and can be used at home—two more benefits.

In general, Chinese massage emphasizes movement and communication. The basic purpose of massage is to restore free movement to the patient's Qi and blood. Chinese massage therapists use a range of techniques to accomplish this: They press, knuckle-roll, squeeze, knead, dig, drag, pluck, tweak, hammer, push, stretch, vibrate, knock, and even tread on the body with their feet. Massage accomplishes its purpose in three ways: it "jump-starts" the activity of Qi and blood; it regulates their movement and disperses stagnation; and it removes external causes of blockage (cold and dampness). Because Chinese practitioners regard massage as affecting all dimensions of the patient's being, they think of it as involving communication between the therapist's Qi and the patient's Qi. In Tui Na massage, the patient is allowed or even encouraged to talk while the therapist is working. This practice often helps the patient to release stored-up feelings.

Tui Na massage takes its name from two Chinese words that mean "lift and press." It requires the controlled use of very deep but constantly moving pressure, repeated hundreds of times. The practitioner pushes hard with the ball of the thumb, then rubs lightly around the area being treated. A therapist using this form of massage might spend as much time on one of the patient's joints or limbs as a Western therapist would spend massaging the entire body. Tui Na is used to treat a wide variety of conditions that would require a team of physiotherapists, chiropractors, and physicians specializing in sports medicine to treat in the West. One Chinese medical book lists more than 140 conditions that can be treated with Tui Na, including disorders of the internal organs as well as sprains, pulled muscles, arthritis, and sciatica (a pain in the lower back and back of the thighs).

Medical Qigong Therapy

Medical Qigong Therapy (MQT) is the final part of TCM, and much like the other aspects of TCM, has been practiced for thousands of years. It is based upon energy (Qi) manipulation methods, both physical and visualized, that are administered by either hands-on techniques (massage and acupressure) or hands-off (distance healing, meditation, and visualization) to purge, tone, and balance the body's

Wei Qi, or energy field. The healing modality most often compared to MQT is Reiki, and while there are some similarities, MQT has many more physical manipulation techniques and a different visualization of energy flow.

Among the techniques of MQT is self-regulation, a technical term for performing Qigong exercises in a medically oriented fashion. Energetic massage, or the act of stimulating the Qi fields by movements of the hands above the patients' body, is also a commonly utilized technique. The entire field of MQT relies, as do the other TCM components, upon the principles established from ancient Taoist philosophy, and an understanding of those principles prepares one to embark upon a lifelong study of TCM.

TCM Diagnosis

You've been suffering from nagging headaches for some time now. Up to this point though, you've endured the pain or taken aspirin and rested when you could. Frequent recurring headaches eventually cause you to worry, however, so you consult your general practitioner. He or she runs a few tests, which rule out anything serious, and prescribes you medication. This works well when you have a headache but doesn't prevent the next one. You go back to your doctor, who refers you to a specialist. Further tests show there's nothing really wrong with you and you're back where you started.

This is a typical scenario for a person visiting a Traditional Chinese Medicine (TCM) practitioner for the first time. Many Western people try acupuncture, for instance, as a last resort after they've been virtually everywhere else. Sometimes their conventional doctor will even suggest it, saying, "Well, at the very least it'll do nothing at all." Or a friend may talk you into it because he or someone he knows had acupuncture and it worked. Desperate for a solution, you find yourself in the waiting room of an acupuncture clinic, contemplating or even fearing what's about to happen.

Although certainly not a cure-all, acupuncture has been used in the Orient for centuries to treat a wide range of acute and chronic conditions. So, what happens from the time you sit down at your initial TCM consultation to when your first treatment is over?

As with your first visit to any healthcare practitioner, the TCM practitioner starts by inquiring about your current complaint. How long have you had it? Is it painful? Is the pain constant or intermittent? Is it sharp or dull? Is the pain fixed in location or does it move around? What aggravates or relieves your pain? What other treatments have you tried or are currently using?

Once the practitioner has noted the necessary details of your complaint, he or she will inquire about other seemingly unrelated aspects of your health. What foods do you eat? Do you sleep well or wake tired or during the night? Are your bowel movements regular? Do you frequently get depressed, frustrated, sad, or angry? What type of work do you do? Do you exercise? Do you smoke? For female patients: Do you experience pain during menstruation? Is the pain before, during, or after your period? Is your cycle regular? What color is your menstrual blood: dark, light pink, red, or brown?

This list is by no means definitive. Different practitioners will inquire about different areas of your health and lifestyle, as they deem necessary. The reason for what, to some, seems like a lot of irrelevant questions, is that TCM is a holistic medicine based on the principle that mind, body, and spirit are interconnected and, therefore, influence one other.

As such, when you consult a TCM practitioner, the bits of information he or she notes about you, that is, your signs and symptoms (s/s), may be likened to the pieces of a puzzle. On their own, there is little meaning, but once assembled, an overall view of your health is established. In TCM, your s/s are grouped into what are known as "patterns of disharmony." These patterns are unique to you, and as a result, your treatment is uniquely tailored to suit your particular condition at that time. The following week when you no doubt feel different, your treatment will change to reflect this.

TCM "patterns of disharmony" are named according to the organ(s) affected and its energetic state. For example, your "patterns" may indicate kidney yin deficiency or liver yang excess or even both. This is also your TCM diagnosis.

To support the practitioner's diagnosis, he or she will feel the radial pulse on each of your wrists, in addition to inspecting your tongue. Tongue and pulse diagnosis are primary diagnostic tools in TCM. The most experienced TCM practitioners can diagnose your condition by these methods alone.

The practitioner, having explained your diagnosis and answered your queries, will proceed with your first treatment, which for the purpose of this section is acupuncture, but may also be massage, herbal therapy, or Medical Qigong Therapy.

Depending on the location and nature of your complaint, certain items of clothing will need to be removed and you will be asked to lie on the treatment table facedown, on your back, or on one side. Exposed body areas are covered with towels. Usually from four to 12 acupuncture points are selected for needling by the practitioner. Commonly needled points are located on the arms below the elbows, the legs below the knees, and along both sides of the spine from the neck to the buttocks. Most practitioners these days use single-use disposable acupuncture needles. Be sure to ask if you're concerned about this.

Once located, each point is swabbed with alcohol before needle insertion. Upon insertion, the practitioner will gently rotate each needle backward and forward and ask you to report any sensations of tingling or warmth around or away from the needle site. These are desired sensations and indicate that the acupuncture point has been correctly located. Generally, needles are left in place for about 20 minutes. Acute and painful conditions usually mean longer treatment time.

All you have to do is lie there and try to relax, although the treatment will often have this effect on you anyway. A commonly reported effect of acupuncture, particularly in people who are tense or in pain, is a feeling of deep relaxation to the extent that many fall asleep during their treatment.

How to Find a TCM Practitioner

When you are searching for a Chinese medicine doctor, the most important factors to consider are the depth of the doctor's training and experience, and your own goals. Remember that Chinese medicine is a participatory process—both you and the practitioner are a team, striving to return you to health.

Training

In order to gain the full benefit of Chinese medicine therapy, the practitioner who administers the treatment(s) should have certifiable training and a good sense of the philosophical basis of Chinese medicine.

The best way to determine if a practitioner meets those standards is to ask a lot of questions about their training, length and scope of practice, specializations, approach to wellness and illness, and understanding of Chinese medical philosophy.

Some Things to Look For

The Taoist system of belief is not some "Johnny Come Lately" that can be cast aside. It is an integral part of Chinese medicine treatments. No Chinese medical therapy can deliver its full healing potential if it is divorced from the philosophical basis of the Tao.

In addition, you want to find a practitioner who is trained in the specific Chinese medicine therapies that you want. Some practitioners are licensed acupuncturists (L.Ac.) but do not offer herbal therapy; there are others who are herbalists but provide no acupuncture; there are licensed acupuncturists who also have training as herbalists; and there are doctors of Oriental medicine (OMD) who provide acupuncture and herbal therapy as well as massage and MQT.

Acupuncturists should be licensed (in states with licensing requirements) or certified. In roughly three-quarters of the states there are state licensing boards, and nationally there is the National Commission for the Certification of Acupuncturists (NCCA).

If you live in a state without a state licensing board, it is important that your acupuncturist have a certificate from the NCCA at the very least. Acupuncture degrees in this country come from accredited schools of acupuncture and Traditional Chinese Medicine schools and colleges. Be aware also that in many states, an M.D. may qualify to practice as an acupuncturist with as little as 200 hours of training, versus the thousands of hours necessary for a L.Ac. or OMD.

Your herbalist (who may also be your acupuncturist) should have either a certificate of training or a long-standing reputation and years of experience. Many schools offer training in herbal medicine, some even offer correspondence courses with a diploma, but be advised that currently there are no independent licensing standards for Chinese herbalists. The NCCA does offer an herbal certification, but it doesn't lead to licensure.

Your Own Goals

You also want to decide if you are looking for a primary care physician, someone to work with your primary care physician, or merely someone who can provide short-term treatment for a specific acute condition.

If you are looking for a primary care physician, I recommend someone who is knowledgeable about all aspects of Chinese medicine and Western medical procedures; someone who will know when to refer you for Western evaluations and testing; and someone who is willing to work with a Western doctor if doing so provides you with the best therapy. They may be difficult to find, however.

To sum up what to look for in a primary care Chinese medicine practitioner:

- Someone who does not make promises to cure disorders and diseases for which there is no cure.

- Someone who understands that there may be many different methods that work for an individual and does not insist that his way is the only right way to go.

- ≈ Someone who "jibes" with you. What interests some people most is ability, and they don't care about personality at all. For others, a more personal relationship is important. You have to make that individual decision.

- ≈ Someone who is able to explain what he is doing from both a Chinese and a Western viewpoint to your satisfaction.

- ≈ A practitioner who is not unreasonably opposed to drug therapy in conjunction with acupuncture or herbal treatment, and who understands (or has access to information concerning) the interactions of drugs and herbs.

In cases of serious illnesses, you want to find a practitioner who understands Western medical terminology and concepts of the immune system, viruses, and cancer, as well as Chinese concepts, if you need treatment for these problems.

If you have HIV, chronic hepatitis, or CFIDS (chronic fatigue immune deficiency syndrome), make sure that the practitioner's attitude is that you can live with this chronic viral infection and that acupuncture and herbs may help you be more successful in that process.

Receiving Treatment

When you select a practitioner and go for treatment, you don't surrender control of your health. Chinese medicine recognizes that we each possess the tools we need to preserve or reclaim good health. The good practitioner simply acts as the guide, helping to coax the body's own defenses to prevent or mend illness and disease.

So, When Do I Get My Black Belt?

Intermediate and Advanced T'ai Chi and Qigong

Intermediate and Advanced T'ai Chi

So, do you get your black belt now?

Sorry, there aren't any belts in T'ai Chi. Or Qigong. Ditto for TCM and meditation.

A little aside about the legendary black belt in martial arts might be in order here. For centuries, belts were used, to paraphrase Mr. Miyagi in *The Karate Kid*, to hold your pants up. There was no need to have any exterior signs of expertise—the only important sign was that you survived up to that point. It was a harsh, cruel world then, with constant warring and political intrigue, and the one sure sign of martial knowledge was that you returned home after the latest war.

When the martial arts began to arrive on American shores, one of the teachers decided that Americans needed some extra motivation to study, because war was something far removed from our everyday experiences. Thus was born the color belts. Over time, more and more colors were added until we arrived at our present-day rainbow of ranks. But perhaps thankfully, T'ai Chi has resisted the urge to confer rank on its practitioners. Ranks of any type tend to set up factions that are envious and jealous of other more advanced factions. In T'ai Chi, we compete with no one but ourselves.

You know what you know, when you know it. Your body will tell you so one day when you're happily practicing your T'ai Chi. You'll be doing the movements so fluidly that your cat will be jealous, and your friends and neighbors will all remark about the "new you." Enjoy that gloating feeling for a while, but realize also that you've only just begun your journey.

Traditional T'ai Chi comes in prepackaged forms, with movements numbering 24, 42, 48, 66, 88, 102, and 108! So learning even the 24-Movement Form can take you up to a year of study, but trust me, the time goes quickly when you are enjoying yourself. And besides the health concerns, that's why you should decide to advance in your studies—because you enjoy T'ai Chi. Because it keeps you limber, but also provides a healthy, fun outlet for you, no matter what your age.

The 24-Movement T'ai Chi Form (also sometimes referred to as the Yang Style Short Form) is a beautiful piece that allows you to gain insight into what traditional T'ai Chi is all about, and provides enough of a challenge to keep your brain working for quite a while. The movements in this form, when properly taught, are *not* difficult, and if you have already tried and practiced the movements in this book, you are well ahead of the other students just starting out in class.

The 42-Movement Form, on the other hand, begins to get a bit more involved, with some tricky transitions and spinning movements. This one is best left until you have learned and are comfortable with the 24 form.

Are you up for a challenge? Then learn the 108-Movement Form, the Granddaddy of all Yang Style T'ai Chi. This one is said to be the original form from the 15th century, so when you learn it, you are learning history! But be prepared to work for that knowledge.

What else is there to explore at this point? Well, you've really only just scratched the surface. Read books, take classes, watch videotapes, explore the Internet— there are so many different avenues of exploration you can follow.

Many of my students started off by taking one of my public classes as a lark— perhaps they were bored or went to support a friend who wanted to try it. But then the bug bit! They came to classes at my school, they started buying books and videotapes, they began taking private lessons with me, and many of them are now T'ai Chi teachers in their own right. Why did they end up this way?

Perhaps it was fate. Perhaps the bug that bit them was more persuasive than they thought. Maybe T'ai Chi reaches something inside of us, something primitive and beautiful that needs to be expressed. Something that that prehistoric caveman might have stumbled upon many moons ago—that one's health is a treasure to be guarded and preserved. What these students found out was that T'ai Chi is an ancient/modern miracle of healing, something you don't come across every day.

Always seek to expand your knowledge of T'ai Chi, no matter what the source. I used to kid my students about the Celebrex commercials on television, and how the commercial was using an age-old modality to sell a brand-new drug. But you know what? That commercial probably did a lot of good for T'ai Chi—it made people aware of the existence of alternative measures for arthritis. I personally gained several new students because of that commercial.

Intermediate and Advanced Qigong

In Qigong, there are also many more paths left to explore, perhaps more so than T'ai Chi. Because Qigong has hundreds, if not thousands, of separate forms, you could spend several lifetimes learning them all. The trick is to find one that is simple enough to learn and remember, but not so hard that it puts your body in jeopardy. There are many that fit the bill—Wild Goose Qigong, Fragrance Qigong, Falun Gong—there are dozens of simple Qigongs to choose from.

I often use an exercise with my Intermediate students where we take the T'ai Chi form (any one will do, really, but we usually choose the 24-Movement Form) and make a Qigong form out of it. This basically involves removing the stepping portion of the form and adding in several repetitions of the arm and waist movements. It's an interesting exercise in that, firstly, you are learning additional movement techniques, and secondly, that you give your brain a new workout! Translating the T'ai Chi moves into Qigong mode requires a good understanding of basic principles as well as the ability to create new moves through that understanding.

Also, with my more advanced students I will often run the Qigong forms backwards. This can take the form of starting with the last movement and proceeding through the form to the very first move (In the 18-Movement Qigong, for example, we start with Press Palms and Calm Down and go backwards all the way to Opening). We also play with mirror-image forms, taking the movements and performing them as if they have been flip-flopped right to left.

What does all this accomplish? Well, most importantly, it amuses *me*! Just kidding....

Again, the benefits of these alterations seem to be that they require a certain mode of thinking to emerge from the students, an ability to create something out of nothing, to look at a problem and see new ways of solving it. It's like aerobics for the brain and the body. They also provide a new twist, literally, to the flexibility aspects of the movements.

Where Do I Go From Here?

As for Taoist philosophy, if this strikes a chord within you, then you certainly can research the history and applications of this wonderful philosophical tool. Remember that people of any faith can benefit from such a study—we are all interconnected on a spiritual level, and it's only the labels that often keep us apart.

Chinese medicine? Another lifelong study. I've been practicing with Chinese herbs for more than 20 years now, and still feel like a beginner. There's always something to learn in this field, no matter how long you study.

With all my years of experience in T'ai Chi, I felt a need to reach out to many more students than I currently could through my present teachings, and this book is the result of that need. Realize that learning a complex movement-based internal art such as T'ai Chi from a book can be a daunting task, but if you're reading this, it probably means that you've stuck it out and at least tried the exercises described here. Congratulations!

Where can you go from here? Well, I would be practicing false modesty if I said that I hope you don't contact me or my publisher, New Page Books, and request more books and videos on T'ai Chi, Qigong, Taoism, and Chinese medicine. I'm ready to teach, as long as you're ready to learn.

There is a saying in the martial arts world: "When the student is ready, the teacher appears." I've always understood this to mean that, given a certain amount of faith in the workings of the universe (Tao), what you need is out there and will find you at the proper time. Your job is to prepare to learn. Remember getting ready for a new year of school when you were a little child? It was a big production—you had to go shopping for new clothes, new pencils and notebooks, and get your hair done—and when the big day came, you were terrified. Well, the same thing happens in T'ai Chi. You can steel yourself to take that class at the YMCA by reading books such as this, watching videos, and talking to your friends, but when you get in that room with those other lost souls, you might start having second thoughts.

But the key to success is to relax and realize that we're all on our own individual path, some of us farther along on that path than others. So we cannot compare ourselves with others. That's one of the most bewitching aspects of studying T'ai Chi—you can be in a studio with 20 other students, but if you are focusing on the movements and your breathing, you lose track of the others. It's just you and the teacher. And even the teacher fades in time….

Always approach your studies with enthusiasm and a thirst for knowledge. Anything less than that will produce inferior results, because we get out of anything only what we put into it. It's so easy to complain about the cold room, or the silly teacher, or the lady next to you in class who just simply cannot stop yakking. We are adaptable beings, in that we can choose to live in one reality or create and inhabit another one. My fondest wish is that you find or create such a reality for yourself through T'ai Chi, and that it brings you joy and good health forever.

Index

About the Author

Sifu ("teacher") Dr. Philip Bonifonte has been involved in T'ai Chi, Qigong, and Traditional Chinese Medicine for more than 33 years. He started his training in T'ai Chi, as well as in several "hard"-style martial arts, at the age of 12 in Chinatown, New York. Subsequently earning black belt rankings in Aikido, Tae kwon do, Hapkido, Judo, and Kenpo, as well as teaching certifications in T'ai Chi, Qigong, Pa Kua, and Hsing-I, he first began teaching private lessons to his students and then started his first school.

In the following years, Sifu Bonifonte owned and operated schools in New York, California, Texas, Florida, and Pennsylvania. He has taught thousands of students to relax and enjoy the benefits of T'ai Chi through his easy-going manner of instruction.

Sifu Bonifonte holds a Ph.D. in Metaphysics from New York University, as well as a Doctor of Oriental Medicine (OMD) degree from the Chinese Hospital of San Francisco. He is also an ordained minister and practicing philosophical counselor.

He currently teaches T'ai Chi at his school, the Chinese Health Institute, in Kingston, Pennsylvania, where he also sees Traditional Chinese Medicine clients for acupuncture, massage, and herbal treatments.

If you would like more information or to contact the author, you can visit his Website: *www.sifuphil.com*, or send an e-mail to: sifuphil@aol.com.

26550493R00121

Made in the USA
Middletown, DE
01 December 2015